EXERCISES IN EPIDEMIOLOGY

EXERCISES IN EPIDEMIOLOGY

Applying Principles and Methods

SECOND EDITION

NOEL S. WEISS

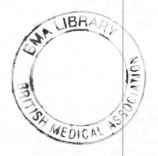

OXFORD
UNIVERSITY PRESS

OXFORD
UNIVERSITY PRESS

Oxford University Press is a department of the University of Oxford. It furthers
the University's objective of excellence in research, scholarship, and education
by publishing worldwide. Oxford is a registered trade mark of Oxford University
Press in the UK and certain other countries.

Published in the United States of America by Oxford University Press
198 Madison Avenue, New York, NY 10016, United States of America.

Library of Congress Cataloging-in-Publication Data
Names: Weiss, Noel S., 1941– author.
Title: Exercises in epidemiology : applying principles and methods / Noel S. Weiss.
Description: Second edition. | Oxford ; New York : Oxford University Press, [2017] |
Includes bibliographical references.
Identifiers: LCCN 2016022295 (print) | LCCN 2016022989 (ebook) |
ISBN 9780190651510 (pbk. : alk. paper) | ISBN 9780190651527 () |
ISBN 9780190651534 ()
Subjects: | MESH: Epidemiologic Methods | Problems and Exercises
Classification: LCC RA652.7 (print) | LCC RA652.7 (ebook) | NLM WA 18.2 |
DDC 614.4—dc23
LC record available at https://lccn.loc.gov/2016022295

9 8 7 6 5 4 3 2 1
Printed by WebCom, Inc., Canada

CONTENTS

INTRODUCTION

There are a *lot* of texts that deal with the principles and methods of epidemiology. I've been a coauthor of one of these myself. All of the texts, to a greater or lesser extent, provide examples of real or hypothetical epidemiologic studies to illustrate a given principle or method. For many (probably most) readers of these books, the examples help to solidify an understanding of the topic at hand.

What the examples do not provide is the opportunity to consider, on one's own, how a particular issue ought to be dealt with, or how a particular question should be addressed. The purpose of this book is to supplement the material contained in the textbooks in such a way that the reader is forced to: (1) identify situations in which the validity or accuracy of a particular design or analytic approach may be limited; and (2) determine how that limitation might be overcome. Such actions are just those that epidemiologists have to take when they are planning research or are reviewing that of others.

The key word in the preceding paragraph is "supplement." The present book cannot stand alone as a means of learning about epidemiology, or even as a means of being introduced to the subject. My hope is that the exercises contained in it can extend the knowledge of students of epidemiology, and equip them more fully to deal with the real world problems and issues that they'll encounter in their professional lives.

This is the second edition of *Exercises in Epidemiology*. As was the case in the first edition, the book is organized into seven chapters, each of which contains a set of questions and answers to those questions. In each chapter the questions from the first edition are placed at the beginning, with the new questions to follow. Any reader who believes a given answer is incomplete (or wrong!) is welcome to communicate with me (nweiss@uw.edu). I would very much appreciate the feedback.

To minimize the likelihood of an ambiguous question being present in this book, or an incomplete or incorrect answer, I enlisted the help of the following persons to review parts of the draft manuscript: Peter Cummings, Paul Doria-Rose, Sarah Lowry, Amanda Phipps, Gaia Pocobelli, Ali Rowhani-Rahbar, Sophie Mayer, Barbara Harding, Alison Rustagi, and Tom Koepsell. Their contributions helped to make the chapters of the book that you are reading better than the draft chapters that they received from me.

EXERCISES IN EPIDEMIOLOGY

CHAPTER 1

Rates and Proportions

EPIDEMIOLOGISTS LOVE denominators. Sometimes we divide the number of numerator events among exposed individuals by the total number of exposed individuals, so that we can calculate the *proportion* of (say) eaters of potato salad at a picnic who were diagnosed with a Salmonella infection during the ensuing 48 hours. At other times, we use a person-time denominator enabling us to calculate the *rate* of (say) lung cancer in persons who have been employed in a given industry. Depending on the question being addressed, we may seek to estimate a proportion or a rate. The accuracy of that proportion or that rate will depend on our ability to measure correctly both numerator and denominator.

Question 1.1 A recent study observed that 1 in 20 persons with cancer later were diagnosed with a second cancer. In the general population, the lifetime probability of being diagnosed with cancer is considerably greater. Is this evidence of immunity developed as a result of the first cancer?

Answer 1.1 This is not necessarily evidence of immunity. What's not being taken into account is the very different denominator for each of the two groups—the amount of person-time at risk. Among cancer patients, person-time begins to accrue as of the date of diagnosis, typically in mid- to late life. In the general population, person-time begins to accrue at birth.

Question 1.2 A study on ovarian cancer observed the following pattern of histologic type and race among its participants.

Race	Type of tumor		Total
	Mucinous	Other	
Caucasian	33 (13%)	225 (87%)	258 (100%)
Asian	55 (27%)	151 (73%)	206 (100%)

The authors concluded that Asian women "had a higher incidence of mucinous tumors" than did Caucasian women. What reservations do you have regarding this conclusion?

Answer 1.2 The observed proportional distribution of histologic type by race could be due to a relatively high incidence rate of mucinous tumors in Asian women, or as well to Asian women having a low rate of other ovarian tumors. For example, the rates below would give rise to the numbers presented in this question:

Race	Type of tumor (rate per 100,000 woman-years)		
	Mucinous	Other	Total
Caucasian	1	6.7	7.7
Asian	1	2.7	3.7

Question 1.3 The following is excerpted from a news item in the *British Medical Journal*:

> The clinical features of more than 1000 patients with lung cancer presenting to 46 UK hospitals have been analyzed. The results showed that women under 65 are particularly at risk of small cell lung cancer—34% presented with this form of the disease compared to 18% of men.

Assume that: (1) the distribution of histologic types of lung cancer in the patients under 65 years in the 46 UK hospitals accurately reflects that of all U.K. lung cancer patients; and (2) the difference between the figure of 34% in women and 18% in men is not due to chance. Under what circumstance could the observed difference *not* be indicative of a difference in the incidence of small cell lung cancer between U.K. men and women under 65 years?

Answer 1.3 The proportional incidence by gender will not be an indication of the absolute incidence if the incidence of non–small cell lung cancer is different in men and women.

For example:

	Men	Women
Small cell cancers (%)	360 (18%)	340 (34%)
Other types	1640	660
Total	2000	1000

In the above example, assuming the numbers of men and women in the population are similar to one another, the rate of small cell lung cancer by gender is nearly identical. The disparity in the *proportional* incidence comes from the disparity in the rates of lung cancer that are not of the small cell type.

Question 1.4 The following statement appeared in a review article:

> In 1996 in the United States, a total of about 34,000 new cases of endometrial cancer occurred, as well as approximately 6,000 deaths from this disease. The case-fatality is approximately 28%.

a. Assuming that the data described in the first sentence are correct, why is it unlikely that the case-fatality from endometrial cancer is truly 28%?
b. Describe a circumstance under which the data in the first sentence *and* a case-fatality of 28% for endometrial cancer in U.S. women could both be true.

Answer 1.4

a. If "equilibrium" exists—in other words, no change in number of cases or case fatality over time—the case fatality among women with endometrial cancer should be 6,000/34,000 = 18%.

b. The 6,000 deaths in 1996 occurred primarily in women diagnosed with endometrial cancer prior to that year. So, if the incidence of endometrial cancer had very recently increased to a large degree, the appropriate denominator for the calculation of case-fatality would be a number much smaller than 34,000 (specifically, 21,429 cases in order to generate a case-fatality of 28%).

Question 1.5 Let's say you've conducted a cohort study to determine some long-term consequences of surgical treatment of patients with cataracts. For 174 patients who underwent surgery and 103 other patients with cataracts who did not, you've used records of the state department of motor vehicles to determine who has been involved in a motor vehicle crash as a driver. From periodic interviews with study subjects, you are able to estimate the number of miles each one has driven during a 2-year follow-up period.

The results of the study are as follows:

Study group	No. of persons	No. of crashes	No. of miles driven
Surgery	174	27	5,677,867
No surgery	103	23	2,569,639

Assume the two groups of patients are exactly comparable with respect to baseline characteristics that predict automobile crash occurrence, including driving behavior, and that no misclassification is present in the study.

a. Estimate the influence of cataract surgery on crash rate while driving.
b. Estimate the overall influence of cataract surgery on the risk of an automobile crash, in other words, that which would include a possible influence of the surgery on driving behavior.

Provide the rationale for your answers.

Answer 1.5

a. The answer is the relative rate based on the number of miles driven

$$\frac{27/5,677,867}{23/2,569,639} = 0.53 - \text{since it allows for the}$$
$$\text{number of driver-miles at risk.}$$

b. Since the number of miles driven seems to have been influenced by the receipt of surgery, the assessment of the aggregate impact should *not* consider this, and the relative risk of $0.69 \left(\dfrac{27/174}{23/103} \right)$ should be used.

Question 1.6 The following is paraphrased from an article in the *British Medical Journal*[1]:

> Although the relative rate of myocardial infarction associated with cigarette smoking is higher in women than in men, smoking may well cause a higher rate of myocardial infraction in men who smoke than in women who smoke.

Under what circumstance could this be true?

Answer 1.6 It could be true if, among nonsmokers, the incidence of myocardial infarction (MI) in men were higher than that in women. For example, assume that in a certain age group the annual incidence of MI was 3 per 1,000 in men and 1 per 1,000 in women. Among men, a relative rate of 2 associated with smoking would produce a rate difference of (2*3/1,000)–3/1,000 = 3/1,000 person-years. Among women, a higher relative rate–3–would produce a rate difference that is smaller than this: (3*1/1,000)–1/1,000 = 2/1,000 person-years.

Question 1.7 The following is excerpted from a letter to the editor of a medical journal:

> We have observed renal cell carcinomas in 6 out of 412 patients with analgesic nephropathy (1.4%), treated over the past 12 years. The incidence of renal cell carcinoma in the general population is 7.5 per 100,000 population per year, so the prevalence found in patients with analgesic nephropathy is highly significant (p <.005).

What additional information on these patients with analgesic nephropathy would be needed in order to better assess the possibility that they are at increased risk of renal cell carcinoma?

Answer 1.7 At the very least, we would need the age-specific person-time at risk for the diagnosis of cancer among participants with analgesic nephropathy. This would permit a comparison of age-adjusted *rates* of renal cell carcinoma between these patients and the general population.

Question 1.8 The Second National Health and Nutrition Examination Survey was a cross-sectional survey conducted from February 1976 to February 1980, with a probability sample of 27,801 persons in the United States.

The following table presents some data obtained in the survey:

Percentage of children 6 months through 4 years with a history of eating unusual substances by selected characteristics: United States, 1976–1980

	No. examined	Percentage with history of eating unusual substances
Blood lead level in micrograms per deciliter:		
30 or more	117	16.2
20–29	503	14.1
Less than 20	1,752	5.2

Earlier studies have shown that elevated blood lead levels (30 µg/dl or higher) are associated with slowed intellectual development in children. At issue in the present analysis is whether eating "unusual" substances (e.g., paint) contributes to elevated blood lead levels.

In U.S. children 6 months through 4 years of age, can you determine the likelihood of having a blood lead level of >30 µg/dl for those with a history of eating unusual substances relative to the likelihood for those with no such history? If yes, what is it? If no, why not?

Answer 1.8

History of eating unusual substances	Blood lead level (microg/dl)		
	≥30	<30	All
Yes	19	162	181
No	98	2,093	2,191
			2,372

$$\text{Relative risk} = \frac{19/181}{98/2,191} = 2.3$$

Question 1.9 The following data were obtained in a very large cohort study conducted in Korea during 1993–2002 that examined potential risk factors (including the prevalence of hepatitis B surface antigen positivity (HbsAg+)) for mortality from hepatocellular carcinoma (HCC).

	No. of HCC deaths	Rate per 100,000 person-years
Men		
HbsAg+	1522	405.2
HbsAg–	734	21.8
Women		
HbsAg+	37	58.4
HbsAg–	9	1.2

a. For men and women, separately, estimate the relative mortality from HCC associated with being HbsAg+, and also the mortality difference.

b. One of the above measures of excess mortality is greater in men; the other greater in women. How can this be?

Answer 1.9

a. Relative mortality

  Men: 405.2/21.8 = 18.6
  Women: 58.4/1.2 = 48.7

Mortality difference (per 100,000 person-years)

  Men: 405.2 − 21.8 = 383.4
  Women: 58.4 − 1.2 = 57.2.

b. The annual mortality from HCC, in the absence of active infection with hepatitis B, differs greatly by sex: 21.8 per 10^5 for men versus 1.2 per 10^5 for women. Thus, an absolute increase in mortality of 57.2 per 10^5 experienced by Korean women is very large in relative terms (relative mortality = 48.7). In men, the larger absolute mortality difference (383.4 per 10^5) is not nearly so large on a ratio scale, since it is superimposed not on a "baseline" mortality rate of 1.2 per 10^5, but on the higher male "baseline" rate of 21.8 per 10^5.

Question 1.10 Black men in the United States have a substantially higher incidence of prostate cancer than U.S. white men. Let's say there's a variant of the androgen receptor gene that's more common in black than white men in the United States—50% versus 30%—that is also associated with a doubling of incidence of prostate cancer in American men of either race.

What would be the relative incidence of prostate cancer, black versus white American men, if the genetic marker were the sole risk factor for this disease that differed between the two races?

Answer 1.10 If x = incidence of prostate cancer in men without the variant genotype, the incidence of prostate cancer in white men would be a weighted average of the incidence in the 70% of men without the variant genotype and the 30% who have it: $7x + .3(2x) = 1.3x$. The incidence in black men would be $.5x + .5(2x) = 1.5x$, because half have the variant genotype and half do not. If, in terms of prostate cancer risk, white and black men were identical save for the prevalence of this genotype, black men would have an incidence that was $1.5x/1.3x = 1.15$ times that of white men.

Question 1.11 You read a magazine article in which a medical columnist has expressed concern that the mean age at which colorectal cancer is diagnosed among Americans who smoke cigarettes and consume alcohol is lower than among their fellow citizens who neither smoke nor drink. Assume that the age distribution is the same between Americans who smoke and drink and those who do not. Must it be true that, among relatively young American adults, the incidence of colorectal cancer is higher in cigarette smokers/alcohol drinkers than in other persons? If yes, why? If not, why not?

Answer 1.11 No. For example, if among *older* persons the incidence of colorectal cancer were relatively low in those who smoked and consumed alcohol, with the incidence among younger persons who smoked and consumed alcohol being the same as that of young abstainers, the mean age of diagnosis of smokers/drinkers also would be lower than that of abstainers.

Question 1.12 The following statement was made in a newspaper article that sought to provide data bearing on the efficacy of seat belts in preventing deaths that occur in automobile crashes:

> Of the 649 people who died in traffic accidents in Washington last year, 55 percent were not wearing seat belts. In those same fatal crashes, 73 percent of people who were belted in survived without serious injury.

Does this statement support the hypothesis that seat belt use saves lives? Explain.

Answer 1.12

	Dead	Alive
Belt	45%	?
No belt	55%	?
Total	100%	100%

The data do not bear on the hypothesis. What is needed instead is information on the percentage of persons who survived these crashes who were unbelted. There would be evidence of efficacy to the extent that this figure was smaller than 55%. Alternatively, one could compare the percentage of *un*belted persons who survived without serious injury to the figure of 73% for belted individuals:

	Dead	Alive	Total
Belt	27%	73%	100%
No belt	?	?	100%

Question 1.13 During a recent decade in the United States, the annual proportion of all women ages 25 to 29 years who gave birth to a first child rose from .031 to .039. In this same decade, however, the annual proportion of childless women ages 25 to 29 years who gave birth to a child fell from .114 to .092. How is it possible that these two trends can be in opposite directions?

Answer 1.13 The numerator for the two proportions is the same, in other words, the annual number of 25- to 29-year-old American women who gave birth to their first child. But the denominator for the second proportion—the number of 25- to 29-year-old childless women—is but a part of the first denominator (all 25- to 29-year-old women). In order for the incidence of first births to have risen overall but to have declined among childless women, it must be true that the fraction of 25- to 29-year-old women who were childless must have risen during the decade. This more than compensated for the declining first-birth incidence in childless women and caused a rise in the first-birth incidence in 25- to 29-year-olds as a whole.

Question 1.14 The rate of suicide among American physicians, relative to the corresponding rate in the population as a whole, varies by gender. Among men, the rate in physicians is 1.5 times higher, whereas among women the corresponding relative rate is 3.0. It turns out that the rate of suicide in American male and female physicians is identical. For American men and women in general, what is the relative rate of suicide in men compared to women?

Answer 1.14

Pm = rate of suicide in male physicians,
Pf = rate of suicide in female physicians.
M = rate of suicide in American men
W = rate of suicide in American women

$$RR, \text{men} = \frac{Pm}{M} = 1.5$$

$$M = \frac{Pm}{1.5}$$

So, for American men in general, their rate of suicide is that of the male physicians divided by 1.5.

$$RR, \text{women} = \frac{Pf}{W} = 3.0$$

$$W = \frac{Pf}{3.0}$$

Similarly, American women have but one-third the rate of suicide of female physicians.

Now, because Pm and Pf are the same (we'll label this rate as P),

$$\frac{M}{W} = \frac{P/1.5}{P/3.0} = \frac{3.0}{1.5} = 2.$$

American men, as a whole, have twice the rate of suicide as American women.

Question 1.15 A study of suicide among men with cancer was conducted in the United States.[2] The goal of the study was to enable health professionals to "be aware of the potential for suicide in cancer patients." Some of the site-specific data are presented below.

Type of cancer	No. of men with cancer	No. of suicides	Suicides per 100 men (95% CI)
Lung	102,940	215	0.21 (0.18–0.24)
Melanoma	19,377	46	0.24 (0.17–0.32)
Thyroid	5,339	14	0.26 (0.14–0.42)

It had been hypothesized that the risk of suicide during any given period of time following diagnosis would be greatest for types of cancer with a poor prognosis (e.g., lung) than types with a good prognosis (e.g., melanoma, thyroid). Do the above data argue against this hypothesis? (Assume that the distribution of demographic characteristics bearing on suicide occurrence is similar across the three types of cancer.)

Answer 1.15 The data do *not* argue against the hypothesis. The analysis fails to consider person-time at risk. Because this is, on average, considerably greater for a man with melanoma or thyroid cancer than for a man with lung cancer, the *rate* of suicide (i.e., number of suicides divided by person-time at risk) in the latter group must be higher than the rate for the other two groups.

Question 1.16 In a study of oral cancer, you observe that 17% of the Hispanic cases are younger than 40 years, as compared to 4.8% of non-Hispanic men with oral cancer ($p < .05$).

Assume that the ascertainment of cases of oral cancer was equally complete in the Hispanic and non-Hispanic men, and that the above difference was not due to chance. Does this finding necessarily imply that in the population under study the risk of developing oral cancer is elevated in Hispanic men under 40 years of age compared to non-Hispanic men of similar age? Explain.

Answer 1.16 No. The age disparity could simply be a reflection of the relatively younger age of Hispanic males in the population under study.

For example:

Age (years)	Hispanic men			Other men		
	No. of cases	Person-years	Incidence per 100,000	No. of cases	Person-years	Incidence per 100,000
<40	17	100,000	17	17	100,000	17
≥40	83	100,000	83	337	406,000	83
% under 40	17%			4.8%		

Or, beyond this, a high proportional incidence of oral cancer in younger Hispanic men could be due to an atypically low absolute incidence in *older* Hispanic men.

For example:

Age (years)	Hispanic men			Other men		
	No. of cases	Person-years	Incidence per 100,000	No. of cases	Person-years	Incidence per 100,000
<40	17	100,000	17	17	100,000	17
≥40	83	100,000	83	337	100,000	337
% under 40	17%			4.8%		

Question 1.17 A population-based case-control study of Guillain-Barré syndrome (a neurological disease) conducted in 1992–1994 in 4 states estimated the risk of this disease to be 1.7 times greater among adults who had received influenza vaccine in the prior 6 weeks than those who had not. The investigators also estimated that the added risk of Guillain-Barré syndrome associated with the receipt of influenza vaccine was about one per million persons during the first 6 weeks after vaccination.

From these data, can you calculate the 6-week incidence among adults in the 4-state population who did *not* receive the vaccine? If yes, what is that incidence? If no, why not?

Answer 1.17 The difference of 1 per million in the 6-week incidence between persons who did (I_e) and did not (I_o) receive the vaccine is $I_e - I_o = 1.7I_o - I_o$. Therefore, $I_o = 1/0.7 = 1.43$ per million.

Question 1.18 The incidence of stomach cancer in country X is 8.0 per 100,000 per year. The incidence rate in nearby country Y, with a similar age-sex-race composition as country X, is 10.0. You are concerned with explaining this difference. You know that 5% of people in country Y drink tea containing suspected carcinogen A, whereas nobody in country X drinks this tea. In order for this to be the sole explanation of the difference in the incidence rates of stomach cancer between the two countries, how strongly must carcinogen-A-tea drinking be associated with stomach cancer?

Answer 1.18 If all the difference were due to ingestion of carcinogen A in tea, the incidence of stomach cancer in country Y could be described as follows:

$$10 = .95(8) + .05t$$

where t = incidence in drinkers of A-containing tea

$$t = \frac{10 - .95(8)}{.05} = 48$$

$$48 / 8 = 6$$

Therefore, a relative risk of 6 (associated with drinking A-containing tea) is required for the whole of the difference in rates between the two countries to be attributable to this exposure.

Question 1.19 During 1993–2001, men at 10 U.S. study centers were invited at random to receive annual PSA screening for 6 years (plus annual digital rectal exams for 4 years; n = 38,343) or no intervention (n = 38,350).[3] Through 10 years from the time of randomization, there were 3,452 cases of prostate cancer diagnosed and 83 deaths from this disease in the group invited for screening, versus 2,974 cases and 75 deaths from prostate cancer among men in the control arm. The investigators noted that, among men diagnosed with prostate cancer in the screening and control arms of the trial, there were 312 and 225 deaths from other causes, respectively, a difference of 87 deaths. They went on to speculate that his latter difference "was possibly associated with over-diagnosis of prostate cancer."

What would be a better approach to quantifying the likelihood of death from causes other than prostate cancer between men who were invited and those who were not invited to be screened?

Answer 1.19 Among men diagnosed with prostate cancer, ideally the *rate* of death from causes other than prostate cancer, not simply the number of such deaths, would be compared: that is, the number of deaths divided by the number of person-years. Even though the sizes of the groups invited and not invited to be screened were nearly identical, the number of men diagnosed with prostate cancer in the former group was larger (by 16%, 3452 vs. 2974), because screening identified a number of malignancies that otherwise would not have been diagnosed during the follow-up period. Failure to take into account the relatively larger number of person-years in the invited men diagnosed with prostate cancer would lead to a falsely high mortality rate in that group.

To the extent that the age distribution of men with screen-detected prostate cancer differed from that of men whose cancer was diagnosed for other reasons, a valid comparison would require age adjustment as well (given the strong association between age and mortality rates).

Question 1.20 The following is excerpted from the Abstract of a report of a cohort study of risk factors for hepatocellular carcinoma.

Chronic hepatitis B virus (HBV) or hepatitis C virus (HCV) infection (OR = 9.10, 95% confidence interval [CI] = 2.10 to 39.50 and OR = 13.36, 95% CI = 4.11 to 43.45, respectively), obesity (OR = 2.13, 95% CI = 1.06 to 4.29), former or current smoking (OR = 1.98, 95% CI = 0.90 to 4.39 and OR = 4.55, 95% CI = 1.90 to 10.91, respectively), and heavy alcohol intake (OR = 1.77, 95% CI = 0.73 to 4.27) were associated with hepatocellular carcinoma. Smoking contributed to almost half of all hepatocellular carcinomas (47.6%), whereas 13.2% and 20.9% were attributable to chronic HBV and HCV infection, respectively. Obesity and heavy alcohol intake contributed 16.1% and 10.2%, respectively. Almost two-thirds (65.7%, 95% CI = 50.6% to 79.3%) of hepatocellular carcinomas can be accounted for by exposure to at least one of these documented risk factors.

Smoking contributed to more hepatocellular carcinomas in this cohort than chronic HBV and HCV infections. Heavy alcohol consumption and obesity also contributed to sizeable fractions of this disease burden. These contributions may be underestimates because persons who took part in the study are likely to be more health conscious than the general population.

a. The authors estimated that "smoking contributed to almost half of all hepatocellular carcinoma (47.6%)." What measure of excess risk are they referring to?

b. How can it be that despite the relative risks associated with hepatitis B and C infection being so high, the percentage of hepatocellular carcinoma attributable to these infections was smaller than that attributable to cigarette smoking?

Answer 1.20

a. Population attributable risk %, that is, the percentage by which the population's incidence could have been reduced had no one in that population smoked.

b. The percentage of cohort members who were cigarette smokers must have been considerably higher than the percentage with either hepatitis B or hepatitis C infection.

Question 1.21 The following abstract (slightly modified) appeared in the *Journal of Urology*.

> *Purpose:* We determined the standardized incidence ratio of testicular cancer in infertile men presenting with an abnormal semen analysis compared to the general population.
>
> *Materials and Methods:* More than 3,800 men presenting with infertility and abnormal semen analysis during a 10-year period were identified. The frequency of testicular tumors detected in these men at the time of their infertility evaluation was compared to the incidence in race- and age-matched controls from the general population during the same period (as reported by the Surveillance, Epidemiology, and End Results [SEER] database).
>
> *Results:* Of 3,847 men with infertility and abnormal semen analysis, 10 (0.3%) were diagnosed with testicular tumors. The SEER database reported an annual incidence of 10.6 cases of testicular cancer (95% CI 10.3–10.8) per 100,000 men of similar age group and racial composition during the same period. The standardized incidence ratio of testicular cancer was 22.9 (95% CI 22.4–23.5) when comparing our infertile group to the control population.
>
> *Conclusions:* Infertile men with abnormal semen analyses have a 20-fold greater incidence of testicular cancer compared to the general population.

What do you believe to be the principal limitation of the comparison made in this study? Explain.

Answer 1.21 The study compared the *prevalence* of testicular cancer in men with infertility (and an abnormal semen analysis) with the annual *incidence* in the population at large. Such a comparison does not permit a meaningful assessment of the possibility of a heightened risk of testicular cancer among infertile men.

Question 1.22 A cohort study sought to determine the incidence of cancer among American children who had undergone renal transplantation. The transplants took place during 1987–2009, with follow-up for cancer occurrence through the end of 2010.

Because of the differences over time in the types of immunosuppression administered to kidney recipients during and soon after transplantation, one of the variables investigated was transplant era. The following data were obtained:

Transplant Era	Cancer Cases		Other Recipients	
	#	%	#	%
1987–1993	18	51	3595	34
1994–2000	9	26	3738	36
2001–2009	7	23	3106	30

A relatively higher percentage of cancer cases were transplanted during the earliest time period (1987–1993), 51% versus 34%. (Assume that the observed difference is not due to chance.) Nonetheless, you are reluctant to conclude from these data that the rate of cancer truly was higher among persons who received a transplant during those years. What is the primary reason for your reluctance?

Answer 1.22 The analysis does not consider person-time at risk. Almost certainly the earliest transplant recipients have been followed the longest. The relatively higher number of person-years they have accrued would have been responsible for this larger proportion of cases even had their annual rate of cancer been identical to that of later transplant cohorts.

Question 1.23 The following is taken from a Commentary (slightly paraphrased) in the *Lancet* (2012;380:1132):

> "The Democratic Republic of Congo has seen its mortality rate of children under age 5 (deaths per 1000 live births) fall from 181 in 1990 to 168 in 2011. Success? No, failure. The total number of deaths among children under age 5 in that country has *increased* from 312,000 in 1990 to 465,000 in 2011, a 49% rise ... Regrettably, the way we talk about child survival—the statistical manipulation of that life into a rate—comes dangerously close to such a deception."

You disagree with the commentator and believe that his approach to judging success or failure would be deceptive. Why?

Answer 1.23 The success or failure of public health and clinical interventions to reduce childhood mortality is gauged by utilizing the data from populations to estimate the likelihood of death in individual children. This entails examining mortality RATES, so as to account (in this instance) for the number of children under age five years. A simple comparison of the number of deaths in a geographic population between two time periods—the comparison favored by the commentator—could be misleading due to an increase in the number of births in that population over time. The larger number of under-five deaths in the Democratic Republic of Congo in 2011 is entirely due to there having been more children under age five years then than there were in 1990.

Question 1.24 The following is paraphrased from a newspaper summary of an article published in a medical journal.

Some 32,154 women were enrolled in a prospective study that sought to assess risk factors for the development of cardiovascular disease at various ages. In women under the age of 30 years, the greatest contributor to the development of heart disease—as measured by the population attributable risk percent (PAR%)—was smoking. But for women in their seventies, it was estimated that physical inactivity was associated with a PAR% almost three times higher than that associated with cigarette smoking, and also more than the PAR% related to hypertension or obesity. The summary concluded by saying that for a woman in her seventies, it appears that physical activity is a particularly important means of reducing her risk of heart disease.

Assume that the data obtained in the study are correct, and that the associations observed are causal ones. Under what circumstance would the high PAR% associated with physical inactivity in women 70 years or older NOT imply that this is a risk factor of particular importance to a given 70+ year-old woman, relative to cigarette smoking, hypertension, and obesity?

Answer 1.24 The size of the PAR% is a function of the relative risk associated with a given exposure AND the frequency of that exposure in the population in question. If in women 70 years and older the prevalence of physical inactivity were very high, even a small excess risk of heart disease associated with it would lead to a high PAR%.

High blood pressure and high body weight could have a more deleterious impact on heart disease risk in a 70+ year-old woman than physical inactivity, but each would have a lower PAR% because their prevalence is considerably smaller than the prevalence of physical inactivity.

The impact of physical inactivity on an individual woman's risk is better assessed by a measure that does not take into account the prevalence of this exposure in the population; for example, the relative risk or attributable risk.

Question 1.25 The nearly 400,000 residential fires that occur annually in the United States constitute a major public health problem—causing substantial mortality and morbidity, and millions of dollars of property loss. Historically and in the recent past, cigarette smoking has been the leading cause of U.S. residential fire mortality, and tobacco smoking accounted for 21% of residential fire deaths in 2000. In 2009, however, the number of residential fire deaths due to heating equipment surpassed the number due to smoking. One state fire marshal hypothesized that this was because of the recession and the high price of heating oil, which may have increased the use of wood-burning stoves and consequently increased the occurrence of deaths from residential fires.

What is a plausible explanation other than an increase in the rate of heating equipment-related residential fire deaths?

Answer 1.25 Another explanation is a decrease in the absolute occurrence of residential fire mortality due to cigarette smoking between 2000 and 2009. (Perhaps the prevalence of smoking declined during 2000–2009.)

Question 1.26 An analysis of U.S. death records revealed that the relative frequency of death from cancer declined from almost 40% of all deaths among persons between 50 and 69 years of age to only 4% among persons more than 100 years of age. The author concluded that people "who survive to ages approaching 100 years are relatively resistant to the causes of death, including cancer, of the majority of people" at younger ages.

You are skeptical regarding the author's interpretation. Why?

Answer 1.26 Rates of death from other causes rise rapidly with increasing age, especially over 100 years. Therefore, the RATE of death from cancer in persons above 100 may even be higher than that in persons at younger ages, and the low PROPORTION of cancer deaths in these older persons due to their very high rate of death from other causes.

(In addition, it is possible that death certificates underreport cancer as a cause of death in 100+ year-olds: cancer in these persons may not get diagnosed as completely as in younger age groups; and, a cancer known to be present in a 100+ year-old may not be cited as reliably as the underlying cause of death.)

CHAPTER 2

Causal Inference

EPIDEMIOLOGISTS' PRIMARY responsibility to society is to provide data relevant to the prevention of disease and injury. We do this by examining the association between disease or injury and potential etiologic factors. When across all relevant epidemiologic studies there does appear to be an association, it is necessary to infer whether that represents cause and effect—preventive measures would be appropriate only when a judgment of cause and effect can be made. To a great extent, the process of distinguishing causal and noncausal associations is subjective: persons may disagree on the relative importance of the various elements that go into such an inference, and on the degree to which those elements are present. However, subjective or not, we cannot escape the need to try to draw causal inferences—an efficient program of prevention depends on our success in correctly distinguishing associations that are causal from those that are not.

Question 2.1 The following is excerpted from an abstract of an article on sudden infant death syndrome[4]:

Objective: To assess the role of parental bedsharing in sudden infant death syndrome (SIDS)-like deaths, this study examines the hypothesis that, compared with other SIDS cases, the age distribution of deaths associated with bedsharing should be lower.

Methods: For 84 SIDS cases in Cleveland, Ohio, 1992 to 1996, age at death, maternal weight, and other risk factors for SIDS were compared for cases grouped according to bedsharing status.

Results: Mean ages at death were 9.1 weeks for 30 bedsharing and 12.7 for 54 nonbedsharing cases.

Conclusion: By demonstrating that among an urban population at high risk for SIDS, bedsharing is strongly associated with a younger age at death, independent of any other factors, this study provides evidence of a relationship between some SIDS-like deaths and parent-infant bedsharing.

In this study, assume that information on bedsharing was completely accurate. What is your primary reservation regarding the authors' assertion that their study "provides evidence of a relationship between some SIDS-like deaths and parental bedsharing"?

Answer 2.1 Parental bedsharing with an infant may simply be an age-related phenomenon: the younger the infant, the more likely the parents are to share a bed with him/her. If so, then bedsharing may have no etiologic relevance to SIDS at any age.

CAUSAL INFERENCE | 59

Question 2.2 Quoted from a magazine of an insurance agency:

> Does your automobile have body damage? Fix it, and you'll significantly reduce your probability of involvement in another traffic mishap. There is a distinct psychological advantage to having even minor auto collision damage repaired as soon as possible. Studies have shown that drivers of newly repaired automobiles tend to drive more defensively than those with unrepaired damage.

Assume that the studies referred to are cohort (follow-up) in type and that they have shown unequivocal differences in the rate of second accidents between persons who did and did not repair the damage resulting from an initial accident. What is your main reservation concerning the conclusion that repairing auto damage influences driving behavior?

Answer 2.2 The association may be due to a third (confounding) factor—persons who choose to have damaged automobiles repaired may drive more defensively than persons who choose not to do so, no matter what the condition of their cars.

Question 2.3 For some time, women taking SSRIs (a class of antidepressant drugs) during pregnancy have been encouraged to stop this medication 14 days prior to the end of the pregnancy, due to concerns about a possible deleterious impact on labor and delivery. A study conducted to examine this issue observed an increased risk of prematurity (<37 weeks gestation) in infants born to mothers who had taken SSRIs and had *not* stopped taking them 14 or more days prior to delivery (women not taking SSRIs during their pregnancy served as the basis for comparison). No corresponding association was seen for discontinuation of SSRIs at least 14 days before delivery.

Even though you have no reason to be concerned with misclassification of exposure or outcome status in this study, or with a difference in risk factors for prematurity at the start of pregnancy between the three categories of women (nonusers of SSRIs, users within the last two weeks of pregnancy, users only prior to the last two weeks of pregnancy), you are concerned that the study does not provide a valid result. What is the basis for your concern?

Answer 2.3 These data may be indicative of a causal rela-tion, but one in the opposite direction. That is, premature delivery in a woman using an SSRI during pregnancy is likely to prevent her from stopping the drug, rather than the reverse.

Question 2.4 The following question pertains to a news item that appeared in a medical journal:

> People screened for lung cancer by spiral CT have accelerated and prolonged quit rates of smoking, regardless of whether the screening shows disease. Researchers found that 1 year after scanning, 14% of smokers had stopped smoking; by contrast, the rate among the general smoking population was 5–7%. The findings suggest that screening is an ideal place to provide cessation messages, say the researchers.

Assume that the difference between the figures of 14% and 5–7% is not due to chance and is not due to differences in demographic characteristics between persons who do and do not receive spiral CT screening. What is an explanation for this difference apart from a genuine impact of attending the screening program on the likelihood of smoking cessation?

Answer 2.4 Due to the likely presence of a great deal of confounding, the data obtained in this study do not have the ability to assess the efficacy of cessation messages to persons who smoke cigarettes. It could be that those smokers who are sufficiently health conscious to receive screening for lung cancer are overrepresented with persons who, apart from any additional health education or advice, are likely to quit during the coming year.

Question 2.5 The following quotation comes from a review of research on diet in relation to levels of serum lipids:

> Many (studies) were limited by having a small number of participants. Diet studies quoted to this day as authoritative had as few as five subjects. If any enduring truth has emerged about human beings and diet, it is that everyone is remarkably different, and studies that don't involve dozens if not hundreds of participants are of extremely limited value.

How is it possible for an epidemiologic study (of any question) that involves fewer than dozens or hundreds of participants to be of more than limited value?

Answer 2.5 I had a professor of neuroanatomy who groused one day in class about a manuscript of his that was not accepted for publication, apparently because the results contained in it were based on but two dogs. He said that if he had just one dog, but could teach it to play the violin, there ought to be no concern with the sample size! If a study has identified a *strong* association (and otherwise has been designed in a way to provide a valid result), it need not be large to document this in a convincing way. For example, it took just 8 cases of vaginal adenocarcinoma and 32 controls to identify an unequivocal association with maternal use of diethylstilbestrol (7 cases and 0 controls had been exposed in utero).

Of course, when associations are not so strong—perhaps in the case of diet in relation to serum lipids—studies of dozens if not hundreds (if not more) participants are needed to document their presence and/or size.

Question 2.6 A study investigated the relationship between a woman's age at first birth and the presence of depression. The study used data from the U.S. National Maternal and Infant Health Survey, a National Center for Health Statistics-sponsored nationally representative survey that selected a stratified systematic sample of 1988 live births from state vital statistics records via a multistage cluster design. Respondents were interviewed in person an average of 17 months after delivery, and the data collected included (among other things) age, race, and the respondent's extent of depressive symptoms in the 4 weeks prior to the interview. On the scale that was used, a score of 16 or higher (out of a possible 60) was the criterion for categorizing a woman as "depressed." This analysis was limited to women who had just delivered their first child.

The following table was presented:

Age, years	% depressed	Odds ratio (95% CI)*
	African-American women	
15–17	48.1	2.7 (1.9, 3.9)
18–19	36.8	1.7 (1.2, 2.5)
25–34	25.3	1.0 (reference)
	White women	
15–17	27.8	2.4 (1.4, 4.1)
18–19	32.9	3.0 (2.0, 4.7)
25–34	13.8	1.0 (reference)

*Adjusted for all relevant confounding variables.

Despite the strong association present in this study, you are reluctant to conclude that giving birth to a child as a teenager is a cause of depression. Why is this?

Answer 2.6

a. The prevalence of depression could be higher in teenagers than in 25- to 34-year-old women even in those without a recent first birth. Thus, the observed association could be related to age per se and not to having had a child at a given age.

and/or

b. Antecedent depression could be more common in women who as teenagers attempt to conceive for the first time (or who fail to prevent conception) than in women who do so at ages 25 to 34.

Question 2.7 In a study conducted among members of a pre-paid health-care plan, an investigator observed that infants of women who had obtained analgesic X from the plan's pharmacy sometime in the year prior to delivery had twice the risk of certain major congenital anomalies compared to the infants of women who did not obtain that drug. Additionally, pregnancies in women who had obtained analgesic X ended in spontaneous abortion 1.8 times more commonly than did pregnancies in women who had not.

The study's findings of increased risk were subsequently criticized because of questions about the accuracy with which infants were classified as exposed or unexposed. Because analgesic X is relatively inexpensive and widely available without prescription, one critic argued that it was likely that some members purchased it outside the health plan. Another critic noted that there was no evidence that the analgesics obtained were actually used during pregnancy. In your judgment, could these factors account for the study's findings, in the absence of a true association? Explain.

Answer 2.7 No. The information bias resulting from these factors would be expected to be nondifferential with regard to the occurrence of a congenital anomaly or spontaneous abortion. This would result in the observed association being spuriously close to the null, rather than away from it.

Question 2.8 A study was conducted among women with either of two types of breast cancer: (1) negative for both estrogen receptor (ER) and progesterone receptor (PR); and (2) all other types combined.[5] The two groups were compared with regard to the use of a statin medication prior to diagnosis. The results were as follows:

	Type of breast cancer	
Stat in use	*ER–/PR–*	*All other*
Yes	34 (11%)	269 (15%)
No	340	1498
	374	1767

a. The difference in prior use of a statin between the two groups of cases was unlikely to be the result of chance (p = .02). The study investigators concluded that statin use could well be related to a reduced incidence of ER–/PR– breast cancer. Assuming that no confounding is present, what is an alternative interpretation of these results?

b. One analysis focused on use of lipophilic statins in relation to type of breast cancer, because of the investigators' concern that prior studies had not accounted for "the confounding effect of combining lipophilic and hydrophilic statins" when examining this question. Assuming that the large majority of women use just one type of statin (lipophilic or hydrophilic), it is likely that the investigators concern was not actually with confounding in those earlier studies, but with another potential source of bias. Which one? Explain?

Answer 2.8

a. It is possible that statin use increases the incidence of breast cancer that is not ER–/PR–.

b. The investigators' concern appears to be with exposure heterogeneity, specifically that an association between the proportional incidence of ER–/PR– breast cancer and lipophilic statin use could be obscured by having included users of hydrophilic statins in the "exposed" category.

Question 2.9 The following data were obtained in a study to evaluate venous thromboembolism risk among women after air travel.

Air travel	Oral contraceptives	# of cases	# of controls	Odds ratio	95% CI
No	No	54	94	1.0	Ref.
No	Yes	95	48	3.5	2.1–5.8
Yes	No	4	5	1.4	0.3–6.8*
Yes	Yes	20	2	17.4	3.9–157.0*

*Exact confidence limits.

The authors noted that they found a marked increase in risk of venous thromboembolism among women who used oral contraceptives and also had recent exposure to air travel, but argued for a cautious interpretation of this finding because of the small number of controls who reported recent air travel and oral contraceptive use. Do you agree that the small number of controls with both exposures argues for a cautious interpretation? Explain.

Answer 2.9 No. Because the lower limit of the confidence interval greatly exceeds 1, chance is an unlikely explanation for the association, notwithstanding the small number of controls with both oral contraceptive use and recent air travel.

Question 2.10 In the United States in 1998, all enriched grains and cereals were required to contain 140 micrograms of folic acid per 100g of grain. Median levels of blood folate among American women of childbearing age rose from 4.8 ng/ml in 1994 to 13.0 ng/ml in 2000.

One of the reasons for the folic acid fortification program was the results of studies (both randomized and nonrandomized) conducted prior to 1998 that documented a large increase in risk of neural tube defects in the offspring of women with low folic acid intake in the year before becoming pregnant and/or blood levels of folic acid at the start of pregnancy. However, a large, multisite, case-control study of neural tube defects in U.S. children born during 1998–2003 failed to identify a difference between mothers of cases and controls with regard to folic acid intake in the year preceding the pregnancy.[6]

Assume that the 1998–2003 study provided a valid result, and that the confidence limits around the risk estimates were so narrow as to exclude the possibility of a true case-control difference of any importance. Why do you believe this null result does *not* detract from the hypothesis that maternal folic acid deficiency is a cause of neural defects in her offspring?

Answer 2.10 It is likely that above a certain threshold of folic acid intake—one effectively reached by all American women after 1997—there is no further reduction in risk of neural tube defects in relation to maternal folic acid intake or blood levels. The inverse association between maternal intake (or levels) and neural tube defects already has been well demonstrated in women below this threshold; the 1998–2003 study simply is unable to address this question in the setting of population-wide high folic acid intake. The cases in the 1998–2003 study no doubt arose via a causal pathway not involving folic acid.

Question 2.11 In an effort to gauge the impact of surgery and radiation therapy on mortality among men with organ-confined prostate cancer that was well or moderately differentiated, a large cohort study was conducted.[7] Beginning one year after diagnosis, all-cause mortality in 65- to 80-year-old American men with this disease who received either surgery or radiation therapy ($n = 32,022$) was 69% that of the 12,608 men who received no definitive treatment, adjusted for tumor and demographic characteristics and for the presence of comorbidity (as assessed in Medicare claims data). For mortality from prostate cancer itself, the corresponding relative risk associated with receipt of active treatment was 0.67.

   a. Based on the adjusted relative risk for all-cause mortality of 0.69 associated with receipt of active treatment for prostate cancer, and assuming that this reduced risk was indeed a result of treatment, how many of the 4,663 deaths in the untreated men in this study's follow-up period might have been prevented had they also been treated?

   b. Perform the same calculation for the 314 deaths from prostate cancer itself, assuming a relative risk associated with receipt of treatment of 0.67.

   c. Assume that classification of cause of death in men with prostate cancer is 100% accurate, and that in truth treatment of prostate cancer does *not* have an impact on mortality from other causes. What do you believe to be the most likely explanation for the difference in the numbers obtained in (a) and (b) above? Why?

Answer 2.11

a. Deaths (all causes) in "observation" group = 4,663
   % potentially averted = 100% – 69% = 31%
   4,663 x .31 = 1,446

b. Deaths from prostate cancer in "observation" group =314 %
   potentially averted = 100% – 67% = 33%
   314 x .33 = 104

c. There were 1,446 – 104 = 1,342 fewer deaths from causes other than prostate cancer in men in the observational group than would have been predicted by the rates in the treatment group. The difference between the observed and expected number must be the result of confounding. Despite the considerable efforts of the authors to nullify confounding (e.g., by eliminating the first year of follow-up postdiagnosis, and by adjusting for demographic characteristics, disease characteristics, and the presence of comorbidity), an inherent mortality disadvantage must have been present in the untreated men.

Question 2.12 The following is an excerpt from an article in the JAMA:

> Age-at-menarche of 38 college female athletes was ascertained and related to the age of initiating training. The 18 premenarche-trained athletes had a mean menarcheal age of 15.1 ± 0.5 years, whereas the 20 postmenarche-trained athletes had a mean menarcheal age of 12.8 ± 0.2 years. Thus, it is apparent that strenuous exercise can delay the onset of menses to a substantial degree.

The authors' choice of comparison is likely to have produced a biased result. Why, and in what direction?

Answer 2.12 The bias results from the fact that the effect being measured—difference in age at menarche—is intertwined with the definition of the groups being compared—pre- versus postmenarche initiation of training. Thus, if a group of girls with age-at-menarche distributed normally about a mean of 13 years all began to train at 13, the mean age at menarche for the postmenarche trained would be <13 years while the mean age at menarche for the premenarche trained would be >13 years. For example:

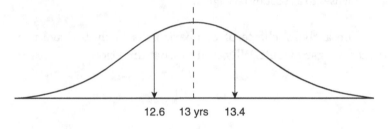

12.6 = Mean age at menarche for "postmenarche trained"
13.0 = Age at which all started training
13.4 = Mean age at menarche for "premenarche trained"

This bias will exaggerate the influence of training in delaying age-at-menarche.

Question 2.13 The following is taken from a 1993 editorial written in response to one of the articles documenting the strong association between prone sleeping position and the incidence of sudden infant death syndrome (SIDS):

"However, these epidemiologic data cannot explain why thousands of babies sleep face down … In other words, the current discussion about potentially amenable risk factors, such as the prone position, may obscure the main goal of SIDS research: understanding the final physiologic pathways that lead to these tragedies and, on the basis of this understanding, finding methods of prevention."

Do you agree that finding methods of prevention of SIDS must await an "understanding of the final physiologic pathways" that lead to this condition? If yes, why? If no, why not?

Answer 2.13 Fortunately, removal of just a single component of a particular causal pathway leading to illness or death can disable that pathway. Therefore, even if we do not know the means by which sleeping in the prone position predisposes to SIDS—"the final physiologic pathways"—the correct inference that this position is a causal factor in some cases allows preventive action(s) to take place. In many parts of the world, parents' choice of the sleeping position of their infants has changed considerably following educational campaigns, and this has been accompanied by a rapid and substantial decline in mortality from SIDS.

Question 2.14 A prospective cohort study in Taiwan observed 40 deaths from liver cancer among men chronically infected with hepatitis B virus, whereas only 0.18 deaths from this cause would have been expected on the basis of the rate in uninfected men. The investigators concluded that the results of their study strengthened the hypothesis that chronic hepatitis B infection is a cause of liver cancer but that, alternately, hepatitis B infection could be a cofactor with another biologic agent.

You take issue with the word "alternately." Why?

Answer, 2.14 It is virtually never the case that a pathogenic exposure is capable of causing disease on its own. Cigarette smoking clearly is a cause of lung cancer, but most cigarette smokers never develop this disease: Something else—one or more genetic or environmental exposures—must have served as a co-factor. Nonetheless, the need for one or more co-factors in order for an exposure to produce its damage in no way detracts from the inference that the exposure served as a cause of that damage. If we can infer that some individuals would not have been damaged had the exposure not been present, we are comfortable labeling that exposure as a cause and regarding it as such—no matter what co-factors were needed.

Question 2.15 The following appeared in an editorial commenting on a randomized trial that had not found evidence of a beneficial impact of a particular intervention on the occurrence of preeclampsia: "The etiology of pre-eclampsia might be multifactorial. Therefore, any single intervention is unlikely to be effective in prevention."

You disagree with the assertion in the second sentence. Why?

Answer 2.15 The assertion is incorrect. Although there may be a number of causal pathways leading to a disease, a single factor may be a component of several frequently occurring pathways (e.g., smoking and lung cancer). Therefore, removal of a single exposure in some instances can have a large impact on the occurrence of a disease.

Question 2.16 The question pertains to the following Abstract, which describes the results of a study that evaluated the impact of a drug administered in an attempt to avert preterm birth:

> **Importance**: In threatened preterm labor, maintenance tocolysis with nifedipine, after an initial course of tocolysis and corticosteroids for 48 hours, may improve perinatal outcome.

> **Objective**: To determine whether maintenance tocolysis with nifedipine will reduce adverse perinatal outcomes due to premature birth.

> **Design, Setting, and Participants**: We conducted a double-blind, placebo-controlled trial performed in 11 perinatal units including all tertiary centers in The Netherlands. From June 2008 to February 2010, women with threatened preterm labor between 26 weeks (plus 0 days) and 32 weeks (plus 2 days) gestation, who had not delivered after 48 hours of tocolysis, and a completed course of corticosteroids, were enrolled. Surviving infants were followed up until 6 months after birth (ended August 2010).

> **Intervention**: Randomization assigned 406 women to maintenance tocolysis with nifedipine orally (80 mg/d; n = 201) or placebo (n = 205) for 12 days. Assigned treatment was masked from investigators, participants, clinicians, and research nurses.

> **Main Outcome Measures**: Primary outcome was a composite of adverse perinatal outcomes (perinatal death, chronic lung disease, neonatal sepsis, intraventricular hemorrhage >grade 2, periventricular leukomalacia >grade 1, or necrotizing enterocolitis). Analyses were completed on an intention-to-treat basis.

Results: Mean (SD) gestational age at randomization was 29.2 (1.7) weeks for both groups. Adverse perinatal outcome was not significantly different between groups: 11.9% (24/201; 95% CI, 7.5%–16.4%) for nifedipine versus 13.7% (28/205; 95% CI, 9.0%–18.4%) for placebo (relative risk, 0.87; 95% CI, 0.53–1.45).

Conclusions and Relevance: In patients with threatened preterm labor, nifedipine-maintained tocolysis did not result in a statistically significant reduction in adverse perinatal outcomes when compared with placebo.

The investigators observed a slightly lower incidence of adverse perinatal outcomes in infants of mothers assigned to receive maintenance tocolysis with nifedipine relative to infants whose mothers received a placebo (11.9% vs. 13.7%, relative risk = 0.87), but this result was well within the limits of chance given no true difference (95% CI 0.53–1.45). Not reported in the Abstract is information on gestational age at delivery. Would this information have been helpful in interpreting the suggestion of a modest beneficial influence of the administration of nifedipine on the occurrence of adverse perinatal outcomes? If yes, why? If not, why not?

Answer 2.16 Yes, the information would have been helpful. Had maintenance tocolysis with nifedipine been associated with a higher gestational age in this study, it would be plausible that the modest observed difference in adverse perinatal outcomes reflected a true modest impact, though one that could not be statistically documented in a study of this size. In fact, the gestational age of infants of mothers in the two groups was identical, arguing that it was not more than chance that the occurrence of adverse outcomes was slightly less frequent in women assigned to the intervention arm of the trial.

Question 2.17 A committee met to review the evidence regarding the possible carcinogenicity of drugs used in the treatment of diabetes. Their conclusion: "There is currently insufficient evidence that anti-hyperglycemic medications are definitively associated with increased cancer risk owing to a lack of data from large-scale randomized trials." Do you concur that in the absence of data from large-scale trials, "definitive" evidence regarding the causes of cancer cannot be gleaned? If yes, why do you concur? If no, why do you not concur?

Answer 2.17 A number of solid inferences regarding the role of medications in causing (or preventing) cancer have been made on the basis of data obtained in nonrandomized studies; for example, adenocarcinoma of the vagina and prenatal exposure to diethylstilbestrol, or endometrial cancer in relation to the use of unopposed estrogen therapy by postmenopausal women. If the association collectively seen across nonrandomized studies is strong enough, and if there is a plausible pharmacologic basis for a relationship, then it would be inappropriate *not* to conclude that a cause–effect relationship is present.

Question 2.18 In a cohort study in Denmark[8] during 1996–2006, the occurrence of autism (A) and autism spectrum disorder (ASD) was examined in relation to use of the drug valproate (V), an agent used by some pregnant women with a history of epilepsy (and by the occasional woman without epilepsy). In this study, a diagnosis of A/ASD (combined) during 4–14 years of follow-up after birth was made in the children of 19.5 per 1000 women with a history of epilepsy who had not used an antiseizure medication during the pregnancy in question. The corresponding occurrence of A/ASD in children born to non-epileptic women was 11.3 per 1000.

In the analysis of their data, the investigators observed that the diagnosis of A/ASD was made in 45.3 per 1000 children of mothers who had taken V during pregnancy, but in only 11.4 per 1000 children of women who had not taken this drug. The investigators also:

- Examined the association between use of V and the occurrence of A/ASD separately in women with and without a history of epilepsy—the association was present in both groups; and
- Examined whether use of antiseizure medications other than valproate was associated with an increase in the occurrence of A/ASD—it was not.

How do the results of each of these latter two analyses bear on the interpretation of the association between the use of V by pregnant women and the occurrence of A/ASD in their children?

Answer 2.18

a. Because a maternal history of epilepsy is a risk factor for A/ASD in her children, and because a maternal history of epilepsy is a strong predictor of use of valproate, the potential for confounding ("by indication") is present here. The presence of an association between maternal use of V and the occurrence of A/ASD in both women who did and did not have a history of epilepsy argues against confounding from this source as the sole basis for the association.

b. The specificity of the association—present only for V and not for other antiseizure medications—also argues that it is the valproate exposure per se, rather than the need for antiseizure treatment, that is responsible for the observed association.

Question 2.19 The presence of the surface antigen of hepatitis B (HbsAg) in a person's blood is indicative of active infection with the hepatitis B virus, but says nothing about when that infection was acquired. In a case-control study in Greece, blood samples from 80 persons newly diagnosed with primary hepatocellular carcinoma (PHC) were obtained and assayed for HbsAg, as well as from 160 controls (persons hospitalized for illnesses other than cancer or liver disease). Also included in the study were HbsAg assays done on blood specimens obtained from 40 persons hospitalized for cancer that was metastatic to the liver from another site. Some 39 of the cases of PHC tested positive for HbsAg, in contrast to 12 of the controls and three of the patients with cancer that was metastatic to the liver.

a. From the data obtained in this study, estimate the risk of PHC in persons seropositive for HbsAg relative to that in other persons.

b. Although one basis for the observed association is an etiologic influence of hepatitis B infection, it is also possible that the presence of an as-yet-undiagnosed cancer allows for a hepatitis B infection to become established in some patients. How does the design of this study go about trying to distinguish between these two hypotheses?

Answer 2.19

a. The relative risk relating HbsAg infection to PHC can be estimated by means of the odds ratio. It is

$$(39/41)/(12/148) = 11.7$$

b. If the presence of cancer in the liver predisposed to hepatitis B infection, it might be expected that a relatively high proportion of persons with a metastatic malignancy in that organ also would be infected with hepatitis B. But this was not what was observed in the study: Only three of 40 such patients were infected, the same percentage (7.5%) as was observed in the controls. The specificity of the association between hepatitis B infection and PHC occurrence, in addition to the very large strength of the association, argues strongly for a causal influence of this virus.

Trichopoulos D, et al. Lancet 1978;2:1217–1219.

CHAPTER 3

Confounding

WHEN THE measured relation between an exposure and the occurrence of disease is distorted by the co-relation of each of these to another exposure or characteristic, we say that confounding is present. Some people, when they learn of an association based on data from one or more nonrandomized studies, do not consider the possibility of confounding, and automatically take the results at face value. Others cannot imagine that it is ever possible to disentangle the influence of one exposure from that of others with which it might be correlated, and so are unwilling to make any inferences from studies in humans that do not entail randomization. Certainly there are nonrandomized studies in which confounding is virtually absent, and others in which it is substantial and uncontrollable. However, most of the time we are in between these extremes, and it is possible to evaluate where confounding might be coming from, gauge its likely magnitude, and even explicitly take it into account in the study design and/or analysis. The questions in this chapter seek to illustrate how all of this can be done in specific circumstances, and also to illustrate more fully just what are the properties of a confounding variable.

Question 3.1 The following questions concern the data presented in the figure below:

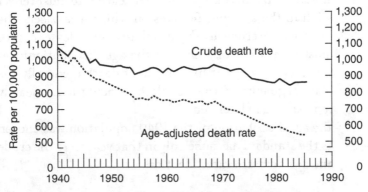

Crude and age-adjusted death rates: United States, 1940–85

a. What is the reason for the increasing disparity between crude and age-adjusted death rates?
b. For purposes of age adjustment, can you tell which population distribution was used as a standard? Why, or why not?

Answer 3.1

a) The sharp fall in the age-adjusted death rate must reflect a fall in the age-specific rates on which it is based. The fact that the crude death rate fell to a much lesser degree must be a result of a shift in the age distribution over time, with groups at higher risk of death (generally the older segments of the population) being more heavily represented in later years.

b) The age distribution of the 1940 population was chosen as the standard, because only in that year were the crude and age-adjusted rates identical.

Question 3.2 The following data are taken from an article on the occurrence of out-of-hospital cardiac arrest in New York City during April 2002-March 2003[9]:

			Incidence per 10,000 person-years	
Race/ethnicity	Population*	No. of cardiac arrests	Crude	Age-Adjusted
Black	1,393,859	1,257	9.0	10.1
Hispanic	1,489,208	636	4.2	6.5
White	2,345,564	1,908	8.1	5.8
Other	829,378	252	3.0	4.8

*18 years and older.

Can you draw any conclusion regarding the difference in age distribution between white and nonwhite residents of New York City ages 18 years and above during 2002–2003? If yes, how would you characterize that difference? If no, why not? (In all demographic subgroups of the population, the incidence of cardiac arrest rises sharply with increasing age.)

Answer 3.2 The white population must be relatively older because once the age difference between groups is accounted for, their rate of out-of-hospital cardiac arrest falls. This can happen only if the white population's age distribution put them at a relatively higher risk than that of members of other segments of the population, in other words, if whites were older on average.

Question 3.3 The following table presents the incidence of hospitalized pneumonia in the United States among persons 65 years and above during two periods of time:

Age (years)	1988–1990		2000–2002	
	Population size	Incidence per 1,000 person-years	Population size	Incidence per 1,000 person-years
65–74	17,506,833	10	18,495,139	12
75–84	9,939,111	21	12,409,949	26
≥85	2,939,646	49	4,413,680	51

An increased incidence was noted in each of the three age groups during 2000–2002 relative to that in 1988–1990. Could confounding by age have distorted the time trends *within* each age group to some degree? If yes, why, and in what manner. If no, why not?

Answer 3.3 Yes, residual confounding by age likely is present to at least some degree in these data, leading to an exaggeration of the true change over time:

a) Rates rise steeply with age.

b) Across the three age categories, there were proportionately more persons in the older group(s) in 2000–2002 than in 1988–1990. Thus, *within* each age group it is likely that the mean age was higher in 2000–2002 than it was earlier. And so, even if the actual rate of pneumonia had not risen at all, it would appear to have done so in each of the three 10-year age groups.

Question 3.4 In a survey of Americans 18 years and older conducted in 2004, 24.1% of white men and 23.9% of black men were current smokers of tobacco. Irrespective of race, the prevalence of tobacco smoking differed little by age, except for a sharp drop in men 65 years and older.

The small difference in current smoking (0.2%) between white and black men noted above does not take into account the fact that in 2004 the average age of white men was somewhat higher. After age adjustment, would you expect the interracial difference to be larger, smaller (or reversed), or unchanged? Why?

Answer 3.4 The adjusted difference will be larger. A greater proportion of white than black American men are in the ≥65-year age group, and these older men have the lowest prevalence of smoking. Removing the age disparity by means of adjustment will allow the higher prevalence of smoking of white men to become more evident.

Question 3.5 The following data come from a Swedish study of children born following in vitro fertilization during 1982–1995.[10] Records of all 26 childhood disability centers in Sweden were reviewed to identify children in this cohort who received services from these centers. In addition, a comparison cohort of children was selected from the entire Swedish Medical Birth Registry so as to be similar to the IVF cohort with respect to sex, year of birth, and hospital of birth.

	Disability	
	Yes	No
All Children		
IVF	101	5,579
Comparison cohort	119	11,241
Singletons only		
IVF	45	3,183
Comparison cohort	115	10,955
Nonsingletons		
IVF	56	2,396
Comparison cohort	4	286

a. What is the cumulative incidence of disability in children conceived by means of IVF relative to that in other children, both adjusted and not adjusted for singleton/nonsingleton birth?

b. Which of the above relative risks addresses the following questions:

   i. What is the impact of IVF on the incidence of disability?

   ii. What is the impact of IVF on the incidence of disability, beyond the impact of IVF to lead to multiple births?

Answer 3.5

a) Crude relative incidence $= \dfrac{101 / 5,680}{119 / 11,360} = 1.70$

Adjusted relative incidence

$$= \frac{(45 \times 11,070 \div 14,298) + (56 \times 290 \div 2,742)}{(115 \times 3,228 \div 14,298) + (4 \times 2,452 \div 2.742)} = 1.38^*$$

b) i. The crude relative incidence. Since multiple pregnancy is a consequence of IVF, it is not appropriate to treat multiple pregnancy as a confounding variable.

ii. The adjusted relative incidence. This tells us how much of an association would remain if, hypothetically, the excess risk of multiple pregnancy associated with IVF could be eliminated.

* Method of Mantel and Haenszel.[11]

Question 3.6 A randomized trial was conducted[12] in which 2,763 women with a history of coronary heart disease were randomly assigned in equal proportion to:

a. a regimen of 0.625 mg/day of conjugated estrogens and 0.25 mg/day of medroxyprogesterone acetate; or
b. a placebo.

During an average follow-up of 4.1 years the incidence of the combined endpoint, myocardial infarction and death from coronary heart disease was identical in the two groups (relative risk = 0.99, 95% CI = 0.80–1.22).

A critic of the study contended that the results may have been confounded, since diagnostic tests to ascertain the extent of coronary and other vascular disease at the outset of this trial were not performed on the study participants. Do you share this concern? If yes, why? If no, why not?

Answer 3.6 Given that this is a randomized trial of 2,763 persons, the treatment and placebo groups would be expected to be extremely similar with respect to their distribution of severity of vascular disease. Failure to have documented that severity in study participants, and thus the failure to adjust for it, should have introduced no bias at all.

Question 3.7 Investigators at the CDC sought to determine the efficacy of the drug zidovudine (AZT) in preventing HIV infection in health-care workers who had sustained a percutaneous exposure (e.g., a needle stick) while caring for patients with AIDS.[13] Among health-care workers with a history of such an exposure, 27 persons who developed HIV infection and a sample of those who remained uninfected were compared with regard to their receipt of AZT soon after the incident.

The analysis suggested that four characteristics of the exposure, or of the patient being cared for, were particularly more common among cases than controls: (a) "Deep" injury, (b) Visible blood on the device that caused the wound in the health-care worker, (c) Injury during a procedure involving a needle in an artery or vein, and (d) Terminal illness in the source patient.

The results of the study pertaining to the receipt of AZT following percutaneous exposure are summarized in the following table:

Number of the other four risk factors	Cases		Controls	
	AZT	No AZT	AZT	No AZT
0	0	0	40	88
1	0	3	51	73
2	2	9	33	22
3, 4	6	7	7	6

Among health-care workers with percutaneous exposure to HIV, estimate the risk of HIV infection in persons who received postexposure AZT relative to the risk in those who did not: a) Adjusted for the number of other risk factors for HIV infection and b) Not adjusted for the other risk factors.

Why do these two estimates differ from one another?

Answer 3.7 From this case-control study, the relative risk associated with AZT can be estimated by the odds ratio (OR). The adjusted OR (calculated here by the method of Mantel and Haenszel) considers only persons with at least one other risk factor, because no case failed to have at least one.

$$\text{Adjusted OR} = \frac{\dfrac{0 \times 73}{127} + \dfrac{2 \times 22}{66} + \dfrac{6 \times 6}{26}}{\dfrac{3 \times 51}{127} + \times \dfrac{9 \times 33}{66} + \dfrac{7 \times 7}{26}} = 0.27$$

$$\text{Crude OR} = \frac{8}{19} \div \frac{131}{189} = 0.61$$

The adjusted OR is well below the null, suggesting a beneficial influence of AZT in blocking transmission of HIV infection. The crude OR is not as low as the adjusted OR, because of the tendency (see the data in the table) for exposed health-care personnel with *other* risk factors for contracting HIV to have received postexposure AZT.

Question 3.8 In white married U.S. males, the annual incidence of prostate cancer is about 1 per 100,000 at ages 35 to 44 years, and about 100 per 100,000 at ages 55 to 64 years.

The following table presents the incidence of cancer of the prostate in white U.S. men, ages 45 to 54 years, in relation to marital status:

Marital status	Rate per 100,000 per year
Married at present	12.5
Never married	11.2
Widowed	20.7

Disregarding the possible role of chance, what do you believe to be the most likely *non*causal explanation for the observed high rate of prostate cancer among widowed men?

Answer 3.8 Because the incidence of prostate cancer rises dramatically with age (1 per 100,000 at 35–44 years and 100 per 100,000 at 55–64 years), the incidence rate is not likely to be uniform within the 45- to 54-year age category. It may be expected that the widowed men within this age category are older on average than the married at present or never-married men, thus accounting for their higher incidence rate. There is residual confounding by age.

Question 3.9 A population-based case-control study of bladder cancer was conducted in a part of the western United States in which some areas have arsenic levels in drinking water that are relatively high (about 100 micrograms per liter).[14] Persons diagnosed with this condition during 1994–2000 were identified through the records of cancer registries serving a 6-county area. Controls under age 65 years were recruited through random digital dialing of phone numbers; controls 65 years and over were obtained through the records of the Health Care Financing Administration. Information concerning a history of living or working in the areas in which arsenic levels were elevated was obtained by means of interviews with the study participants, as was information on potential confounding factors.

On average, income levels in cases were lower than those of controls.

In discussing their findings, the authors acknowledged this imbalance, and suggested it was "likely related to the increased participation rates among [potential controls] in higher socioeconomic brackets." Nonetheless, they concluded, "Other studies have shown little or no association between socioeconomic status and bladder cancer, suggesting that this variable is not likely to act as a substantial confounder."

In this study, do you believe it would be possible for "annual income" to be a confounding variable when assessing the potential association between arsenic in drinking water and the incidence of bladder cancer? If yes, under what circumstance? If no, why not? (Assume that income level has been measured without error.)

Answer 3.9 Income will be a confounder if it is related, positively or negatively, to ingestion of arsenic. Income is already related to case/control status, probably by virtue of differences in level of participation across socioeconomic strata (as the authors suggest). The fact that income level is not truly a risk factor for bladder cancer in the population at large is irrelevant, given the case/control disparity in the distribution of income in *this* study.

Question 3.10 The following table contains data from a New Zealand study in which automobiles involved in crashes and a random sample of other automobiles were compared for color.[15]

Association of car color with car crash injury in Auckland

Car color	No. (%) of cases (n = 567)	No. (%) of controls (n = 588)	Univariate odds ratio	Multivariable odds ratio*
White	145 (25.6)	146 (25.9)	1	1
Yellow	31 (5.5)	15 (2.8)	2.0 (1.0 to 4.0)	0.8 (0.3 to 2.3)
Grey	52 (9.2)	61 (10.0)	0.9 (0.6 to 1.5)	0.6 (0.3 to 1.3)
Black	36 (6.4)	34 (5.5)	1.2 (0.7 to 2.0)	2.0 (1.0 to 4.2)
Blue	91 (16.1)	96 (17.4)	0.9 (0.6 to 1.4)	0.9 (0.5 to 1.6)
Red	85 (15.0)	82 (13.3)	1.1 (0.7 to 1.8)	0.7 (0.4 to 1.4)
Green	42 (7.4)	44 (7.0)	1.1 (0.6 to 1.8)	1.8 (1.0 to 3.6)
Brown	55 (9.7)	49 (6.8)	1.4 (0.8 to 2.5)	2.1 (1.1 to 4.2)
Silver	30 (5.3)	61 (11.3)	0.5 (0.3 to 0.8)	0.4 (0.2 to 0.9)

*Adjusted for driver's age, ethnicity, alcohol consumption in past 6 hours, seat belt use, vehicle speed, average driving time each week, driving license status, vehicle insurance status, and weather.

From the information contained in the table, which one of the following statements do you believe to be true? Explain your answer.

   a) On the basis of their age, ethnicity, alcohol consumption, and so forth (see footnote to the table), drivers of black or brown cars in Auckland during 1998–1999 tended to be at *higher* risk of a car crash injury than drivers of white cars.

   b) On the basis of their age, ethnicity, alcohol consumption, and so forth (see footnote to the table), drivers of black or brown cars in Auckland during 1998–1999 tended to be at lower risk of a car crash injury than drivers of white cars.

   c) From the data presented, no inferences can be made from these data regarding the underlying differences in risk between drivers of black/brown versus white cars.

Answer 3.10 The correct answer is (b). Since adjustment for the characteristics listed in the footnote led to an increase in the OR associated with driving a black or brown car, the underlying risk of a car crash injury must have been low relative to drivers of white cars.

Question 3.11 The following table is from an article that describes the prevalence at birth of a particular congenital malformation in Ontario, Canada, before and after a program of folate fortification of cereal grain products was begun in January, 1998[16]:

	Before fortification	After fortification	Crude prevalence ratio (95% CI)	Age-adjusted prevalence ratio (95% CI)
Length of observation (months)	48	29		
Maternal age (mean, SD) (years)	30.1 (0.16)	30.9 (0.081)		
Number of women	218,977	117,986		
Number of women with an affected child	248	69		
Prevalence (per 1,000 infants)	1.13	0.58	0.52 (0.40–0.67)	0.62 (0.46–0.83)

From the data presented in the table, what can be concluded regarding an association between maternal age and the occurrence of this malformation? Explain your answer.

a) On average, the risk rises with increasing maternal age.
b) On average, the risk falls with increasing maternal age.
c) The risk is unaffected by maternal age.
d) No conclusion can be drawn about a relation of maternal age to the prevalence of the malformation from these data.

Answer 3.11 The crude and age-adjusted relative risks associated with being born after the introduction of fortification differ, so maternal age must be related to the occurrence of the malformation. And, since we know that:

a) women in the latter time period were, on average, older than those in the earlier period;

and

b) adjustment for maternal age made the prevalence ratio rise,

older women must be a lower risk age group. The correct answer is (b).

Question 3.12 The following is an excerpt from an article, "Cancer beats a retreat," that appeared in a 1998 issue of *US News and World Report*. It dealt with recent declines in cancer incidence rates in the United States.

> The researchers acknowledge that the cancer war might not be doing as well as the new data suggest. They adjusted their numbers on the basis of the age of the U.S. population in 1970, a widely used standard in cancer studies. However, the population has aged in the past 25 years. Since cancer disproportionately strikes older people, using a current standard might yield less encouraging results.

Is it possible that using the age distribution of the U.S. population in 1990 as a standard "might yield less encouraging results" than using the 1970 population? If so, how could this occur? If not, why not?

Answer 3.12 The use of the 1990 U.S. population as a standard (which gives more weight to the rates in older age groups) would tend to give a relatively smaller estimate of the declining rate only if the size of the decline were smaller in older than in younger persons.

Question 3.13 The following is excerpted from a letter to the editor of a medical journal:

> There is a sharp contrast in the consistency of success in studies that have sought genotype-phenotype associations in animals and in humans. For example, animal models of depression and anxiety disorders have consistently demonstrated genotype-phenotype associations. By contrast, a recent genome-wide association study (GWAS) of depression found no significant associations. One central difference between these 2 research approaches lies in control over potentially relevant environmental exposures. These exposures are effectively randomized in animal models, but such control is absent from observational human gene-hunting studies.

Assume that the genome-wide association studies were conducted in racially homogeneous populations. Do you agree that the lack of randomization in these studies is likely to be responsible for the difference between their results and those obtained in studies conducted in other species? If yes, why? If no, why not?

Answer 3.13 No. Whatever environmental exposures are related to the development of depression and anxiety disorders in human beings, these almost certainly do not bear on a person's genotype. Given the likely absence of confounding, the lack of randomization of genotype in human studies of depression should not affect the validity of the results obtained.

Question 3.14 The data presented in the following table come from in-person interviews of random samples of the U.S. population ages 19 years and above. They indicate that the prevalence of cigarette smoking in 2008 was greater among American Indian/Alaska Native persons than among non-Hispanic whites. The data are not adjusted for age, however, and the proportion of American Indians/Alaska Natives over 64 years of age in those years was smaller than the corresponding proportion of non-Hispanic whites. If age adjustment were to be done, would you expect the difference in smoking prevalence between these two demographic subgroups to increase, shrink, or remain the same? Explain.

Percentage of persons aged ≥18 years who were current cigarette smokers, by sex, race/ethnicity, and age—National Health Interview Survey, United States 2008

Characteristic	Men (n = 9,387) % (95% CI)	Women (n = 12,138) % (95% CI)
Race/Ethnicity		
White, non-Hispanic	23.5 (22.2–24.9)	20.6 (19.3–21.9)
American Indian/ Alaska Native	42.3 (27.4–57.2)	22.4 (12.5–32.3)
Age (yrs)		
18–24	23.7 (20.3–27.1)	19.0 (16.2–21.8)
25–44	26.4 (24.5–28.2)	21.1 (19.5–22.7)
45–64	24.8 (22.8–26.7)	20.5 (18.9–22.1)
≥65	10.6 (8.8–12.3)	8.4 (7.1–9.6)

Answer 3.14 The difference would be expected to shrink. Younger Americans tend to be current smokers more than older ones (see table), and American Indians/Alaska Natives tend to be younger than whites. Thus, a part of the difference in smoking prevalence is attributable to age alone, and that part would disappear with age adjustment.

Question 3.15 The following appeared in the November 13, 1999, issue of *Lancet*:

> The general health of the East German population was below the standard of their Western counterparts despite an emphasis on public health. In 1991, life expectancy was 3.2 years shorter in men (69.9 years) and 2.3 years in women (77.2 years) than in West Germans. Mortality in 1991 also showed important differences: 1324 per 100,000 population in East German women, 1215 in men compared with 1149 in West German women and 1061 in men.

In trying to determine whether the risk of death differed between East and West Germans in 1991, you'd be loath to use the mortality rates provided in this article. Why do you believe they might be misleading?

Answer 3.15 The mortality rates for 1991, higher in women than in men in both populations, must not be age-adjusted. (We know this because the greater life expectancy in German women than German men must be a result of the age-specific mortality among women being *low* relative to that of men.) Therefore, if the East German population had been older, on average, than the West German population, some or all of the difference in the crude mortality rates could be due to confounding by age.

Question 3.16 I came across the following statement (and data) in a draft of a master's thesis a *long* time ago. Can you think of a reason that the observed association between marital status and suicide is almost certainly greatly overestimated?

In general, suicide is less frequent among the married—except for the young married population. As the table indicates, in the under-20 age group, suicide rates are higher in married or divorced persons than in single persons. Explanations for this phenomenon may be a desire to escape unsatisfactory home conditions or pregnancy resulting in an unplanned, unhappy marriage.

Death rates from suicide by marital status and sex, persons less than 20 years of age: United States, 1949–1951

	Total	Single	Married	Divorced
White males	0.9	0.9	6.2	14.5
White females	0.4	0.3	3.1	13.8

Answer 3.16 There is an unusually great degree of confounding by age here. Persons at the upper end of the 0- to 20-year age groups are the ones relatively most likely to get married (and divorced) and (irrespective of marital status) to commit suicide.

Question 3.17 The following data describe the occurrence of primary cesarean delivery (i.e., in women with no prior cesarean delivery), expressed as a percentage of all live births, in the United States in 1990:

	Total	Under 20 years	20–24 years	25–29 years	30–34 years	35–39 years	40–49 years
				Age of mother			
All births	16.0	14.7	15.0	16.0	16.5	19.0	23.5
1st	24.6	16.9	22.6	27.1	32.2	39.2	46.9
2nd	8.9	6.8	7.3	8.7	10.4	13.6	20.1
3rd	8.4	6.3	6.5	7.7	9.0	12.0	18.1
4th and over	8.8	7.6	6.8	7.4	8.8	11.2	15.1

There is generally a 2- to 3-fold difference in the proportion of cesarean deliveries between the youngest and the oldest categories of maternal age within individual categories of live birth order. However, the difference is considerably smaller—14.7 percent versus 23.5 percent—when the comparison is made for all birth orders combined.

What do you believe to be the explanation for the relative difference in the frequency of cesarean delivery across maternal age being so much smaller when examined overall than within individual birth order categories? Why?

Answer 3.17 There is confounding by birth order: (a) at any maternal age, first births are associated with relatively high percentage of cesarean deliveries; (b) young mothers, relative to older ones, would be expected to be in the lower birth orders, and on that basis alone would be at increased risk of cesarean section. The confounding attenuates to some degree the very strong association seen in the birth-order specific results.

Question 3.18 In a case-control study that was based on information obtained from spouses, a history of high-intensity leisure-time physical activity (LTPA) during the prior year was associated with a reduced risk of primary cardiac arrest.[17] Relative to the risk in persons with light or no LTPA, that in persons with high-intensity activity was 0.19; after adjusting for age, smoking, education, diabetes, hypertension and self-reported health status ("fair," "good," "excellent," or "very good"), the corresponding relative risk was 0.36.

There was a case-control difference in self-reported health status, and it is reasonable to assume that adjustment for this variable explained at least some of the difference between the unadjusted and adjusted odds ratios associated with high-intensity LTPA. However, health status is difficult to assess from interview data alone, so some subjects were probably misclassified on this variable. Had no misclassification been present, what would you predict the adjusted odds ratio associated with high intensity LTPA to be?

a. 0.36
b. Greater than 0.36
c. Less than 0.36
d. No prediction is possible.

Explain your answer.

Answer 3.18 Inaccurate measurement of a confounding variable will give rise to an adjusted risk estimate that is spuriously close to the unadjusted one. So, more complete adjustment for self-reported health status would be expected to lead to a relative risk associated with high LTPA that is greater than 0.36.

Question 3.19 Investigators in Australia surveyed 202 pregnant women who were undergoing abortion who were using oral contraceptives (OCs) when they became pregnant. Among other things, the investigators gathered information on type of OC used by these 202 women, in comparison with the types of OCs used by all OC users in Australia. They were specifically interested in pregnancies among women using triphasic OCs. They presented the following results:

	Abortion-seeking OC users	All Australian OC users
Mean age	23 years	30 years
Type OC used		
Triphasic	52%	42%
Monophasic		
30 microgram ethinylestradiol	27.2%	29.2%
50 microgram ethinylestradiol	7.9%	13.2%
Norethisterone	9.4%	9.0%
Progestin-only	3.5%	6.2%

The investigators found that triphasic OC use was more common (P <0.01) in OC users seeking abortion than would be expected based on the national usage. They concluded that triphasic OCs were more likely than other OCs to increase the risk of inadvertent pregnancy (and they hypothesized this was because they have a smaller margin of safety due to decreased progestin content).

You are concerned that the age difference between the two groups above could be distorting the results. Under what circumstance would this be so?

Answer 3.19 These data indicate that OC users seeking abortion are younger than OC users overall. If young age is associated with an increased risk of abortion (either because of a greater risk of pregnancy, or among pregnant women, a greater use of induced abortion) and if younger OC users tend to use triphasic preparations relatively more than older women do, it is possible that there is no true association between triphasic OC use and inadvertent pregnancy. Information on the type of OC use, by age, is necessary to determine if this is the case.

Question 3.20 A case-control study of the relationship between asthma and a history of pertussis vaccination among children (2 years of age) was carried out in one community. Although overall participation was good, not all parents of cases and controls could be interviewed. A difference in the percentage interviewed based on case/control status and on day care enrollment was noted. Only 63% of control parents with a child enrolled in day care could be interviewed, versus 82% of control parents with a child who was not enrolled in day care. In all, 93% of case parents were interviewed, a percentage that was the same for parents of children who were and were not enrolled in day care.

In this study, under what circumstance would "enrollment in day care" confound the association between asthma and pertussis vaccination?

Answer 3.20 Because there was differential case-control response by day care enrollment status, day care enrollment would be a confounder if it were also associated with pertussis vaccination status.

Question 3.21 A case-control study of breast cancer in relation to prior use of postmenopausal hormones was conducted among American women enrolled in a network of health insurance plans.[18] Women who were newly diagnosed with breast cancer and who had been enrolled for at least 2 years prior to that date comprised the case group.

For each case, four women were selected as controls, matched on year of birth and enrollment status as of the time of the case's diagnosis (and for the 2 years prior to that time).

Data on hormone use were obtained from paid claims for pharmaceuticals. While a similar proportion of cases and controls had taken estrogen alone prior to the time of the cases' diagnoses (odds ratio = 0.96, referent category being hormone nonusers), a higher portion of cases than controls had taken combined estrogen-progestin therapy (odds ratio = 1.44, referent category being hormone nonusers).

The information available on study subjects did not include whether they had a history of bilateral oophorectomy. Such a history is associated with a reduced risk of breast cancer. If a woman has not undergone bilateral oophorectomy and is prescribed hormone therapy, generally that therapy will be in the form of a combined estrogen-progestin regimen. Women whose ovaries have been removed generally will be given estrogen alone.

Is there reason to believe that the two odds ratios obtained are biased due to the investigators' inability to adjust for a history of bilateral oophorectomy? If yes, why, and in which direction? If no, why not?

Answer 3.21 The inability to adjust for a history of bilateral oophorectomy will lead to bias (confounding), at least to some degree. Based on their absence of ovarian tissue, the users of estrogen alone are a low-risk group for breast cancer: therefore, the odds ratio associated with use of estrogen alone that was obtained in this study is spuriously low. In contrast, users of combined therapy have an inherently elevated risk, since they do have intact ovaries. As a result, this study's odds ratio associated with receipt of hormone therapy is likely to be falsely high.

Question 3.22 Based on the figure below, which one of the following statements is correct for American women giving birth during 1979–1982:

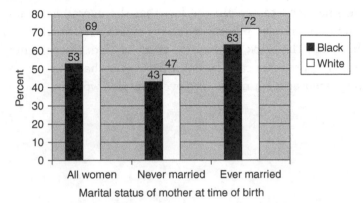

Percentage of mothers receiving prenatal care in the first trimester, by race and marital status: United States, 1979-1982

a) A greater proportion of white than black mothers had never been married.

b) A greater proportion of black than white mothers had never been married.

c) An equal proportion of black and white mothers had never been married.

d) From the data provided, no conclusion as to the marital status distribution of white and black mothers is possible.

Explain your answer.

Answer 3.22 The correct answer is (b). Overall, 69% of white women received prenatal care, a weighted average of the figures of 47% for never-married women and 72% for ever-married women. The preponderance of these women must have been ever-married,* to explain the fact that the overall percentage and never-married percentage are so similar. In contrast, only about half the black women had ever married: the percentage receiving prenatal care overall—53%—lies halfway between the percentages for never- and ever-married women.

---

* x = proportion of white women who were ever married
  $72x + 47 (1-x) = 69$
  $x = 0.88$

Question 3.23 The following data come from a 1975 survey of a representative sample of about 140,000 persons from the United States population:

Age (years)	% cigarette smokers	
	Male	Female
21–24	41.3	34.0
25–34	43.9	35.4
35–44	47.1	36.4
45–54	41.1	32.8
55–64	33.7	25.9
65–74	24.2	7.1

Marital Status	% cigarette smokers	
	Male	Female
Married	38.3	28.3
Single	37.5	30.6
Divorced or separated	60.1	50.0
Widowed	35.7	19.3

From these data, can you conclude that there is an association, beyond that which could be explained on the basis of age: (a) between smoking and widowhood among females? (b) among persons of both sexes, between smoking and being divorced or separated? (No calculations are required.)

Answer 3.23

a) Widowed women are likely to be considerably older, on average, than other women, and (at the time the data were collected) older women were less often cigarette smokers than younger women. Thus, it is possible that after controlling for age, widows may not have had a smaller proportion of cigarette smokers than women in the other marital status categories.

b) The frequency of cigarette smoking among divorced/ separated persons was high—50%–60%—relative to that of any age groups in the population as a whole. No matter what the age distribution of divorced/separated persons, a prevalence of cigarette smoking of 50%–60% cannot be explained solely by of an overrepresentation of a particular age group. An association beyond that which could be explained by age must have been present.

Question 3.24 This question is based on the following (slightly paraphrased) abstract[19]:

> *Background.* Among women pregnant for the second time, the risk of pre-eclampsia is lower than in their first pregnancy, but not if the mother has a new partner for the second pregnancy. One explanation is that the risk is reduced with repeated maternal exposure and adaptation to specific antigens from the same partner. However, the difference in risk might instead be explained by the interval between births.
>
> *Methods.* We used data from the Medical Birth Registry of Norway, a population-based registry that includes births that occurred between 1967 and 1998. We studied 551,478 women who had two or more singleton deliveries.
>
> *Results.* The risk of pre-eclampsia in a second pregnancy was directly related to the time that had elapsed since the preceding delivery, and when the interbirth interval was 10 years or more, the risk approximated that among women pregnant for the first time. In unadjusted analyses, a second pregnancy involving a new partner was associated with higher risk of pre-eclampsia than a second pregnancy with the same partner, but after adjustment for the interbirth interval, the difference in risk of pre-eclampsia was reduced.

From the foregoing, what can be concluded about the relation between interbirth interval and the presence of a new partner? Explain your answer.

a) Women with new partners tended to have a shorter interbirth interval than women with the same partner.

b) Women with new partners tended to have a relatively longer interbirth interval.

c) Women with or without new partners had, on average, the same interbirth interval.

d) Nothing can be concluded about a possible association between interbirth interval and the presence of a new partner.

Answer 3.24 The correct answer is (b). The presence of a new partner must be associated with a longer interbirth interval. The crude elevated risk for pre-eclampsia present in women with new partners was diminished once adjustment was made for interbirth interval. Therefore, since long interbirth intervals are associated with high risk, these must have been relatively more common in women with new partners.

Question 3.25 It is well documented that the presence of nausea and vomiting in the first trimester of pregnancy is associated with a reduced risk of spontaneous abortion in that pregnancy. Imagine a cohort study in which the occurrence of spontaneous abortion is compared between pregnant women who do and do not take an anti-emetic drug during the first trimester, a study in which no information is available on the presence of nausea or vomiting. Assume that truly the drug produces no altered risk of spontaneous abortion. Would you expect the observed relative risk associated with use to be:

(a) 1.0
(b) Less than 1.0
(c) Greater than 1.0

Explain.

Answer 3.25 Because of confounding, the observed relative risk would be expected to be below 1.0: Women who take the drug are inherently at a reduced risk of sustaining a spontaneous abortion, due to physiologic changes that also lead them to have nausea or vomiting. As an example, a study of pregnancy outcomes in Danish women during 1997–2011[21] observed users of the anti-emetic drug metoclopramide to have had but 35% the number of spontaneous abortions that would have been expected on the basis of the incidence among pregnant nonusers of anti-emetic drugs.

Question 3.26 The following (slightly paraphrased) opinion was expressed in a letter to the editor of a medical journal (JAMA 2009;302:1859).

There is a sharp contrast in the consistency of success in studies that have sought genotype–phenotype associations in animals and in humans. For example, animal models of depression and anxiety disorders consistently have demonstrated genotype–phenotype associations. By contrast, a recent genome-wide association study (GWAS) of depression found no significant associations. One central difference between these two research approaches lies in control over potentially relevant environmental exposures. These exposures are effectively held constant in studies using animal models, but such control is absent from observational human gene-hunting studies.

Assume that the genome-wide association studies were conducted in racially homogeneous populations. Do you agree that the lack of control of environmental exposures in these studies is likely to be responsible for the difference between their results and those obtained in studies conducted in other species? If yes, why? If no, why not?

Answer 3.26 You disagree. Whatever environmental exposures are related to the development of depression and anxiety disorders in human beings, these almost certainly do not bear on a person's genotype, and, therefore, cannot be expected to confound the association between genotype and depression and/or anxiety. The lack of control of environmental exposures in human studies of depression or anxiety in relation to genotype should not affect the validity of the results obtained.

Question 3.27 In a cohort study of women ≥ 35 years of age, a sharp gradient of increasing risk of femoral fracture was observed in relation to progressively decreasing bone mineral density. Despite the rapid rise in the incidence of femoral fracture with increasing age, the investigators chose not to control for age in this analysis because bone density measurements "are strongly correlated with age . . . so [prior] studies that used control women matched on age have to some extent matched on bone density as well."

What do you believe is the principal downside to the authors' decision to not control for age? In what direction would it have distorted the measured association between bone mineral density and risk of femoral fracture?

Answer 3.27 There are likely to be other risk factors for femoral fracture that also are associated with age—for example, decreased motor coordination, muscle weakness, and impaired balance. By not controlling for age, the effects of these other characteristics are being mixed with the effect of low bone-mineral density, leading to an exaggeration of the inverse density–fracture association.

Question 3.28 In a European cohort study, 126,920 women were interviewed and then monitored for cancer incidence for nine years. Among those with at least one intact ovary at baseline, the subsequent incidence of ovarian cancer was 19% higher in women who reported current use of postmenopausal hormone therapy than in those who had never used such therapy. However, prior use of oral contraceptives (OCs) was considerably more common in current users (62.1%) than in never users (37.6%), and use of oral contraceptives is known to decrease the risk of ovarian cancer.

a. When estimating the risk of ovarian cancer associated with use of postmenopausal hormones, would it be appropriate to adjust for prior use of oral contraceptives? Explain.

b. If adjustment were done, would you expect the resulting relative risk to be lower than, the same as, or higher than 1.19? Why?

154 | EXERCISES IN EPIDEMIOLOGY

Answer 3.28

    a. Yes, it would be appropriate to adjust for OC use. Such use is associated with both exposure and outcome, and is not a consequence of either.

    b. The OC-adjusted relative risk will be higher than the crude one. Because a comparatively high proportion of women receiving postmenopausal hormone therapy had previously used OCs, they were at a reduced risk of developing ovarian cancer. If that advantage were to be negated—by adjustment for OC use—their relative incidence of ovarian cancer would rise, increasing the risk relative to that in nonusers of postmenopausal hormones.

Question 3.29 Based on the information provided below, can you predict the direction of the change (if any) in the association between weight cycling (as defined) and cancer X among women who participated in the study once adjustment for body mass index has taken place? If so, what is that direction, and how were you able to determine it? If not, why not?

> **Background:** Obesity, as measured by body mass index (BMI), is an established risk factor for cancer X in postmenopausal women. Weight cycling, which consists of repeated cycles of weight loss followed by regain, occurs relatively more frequently in overweight and obese women. It is unclear whether weight cycling is associated with risk of cancer X independent of BMI.

> **Methods:** This analysis included 38,148 postmenopausal women enrolled in the study, of whom 559 were diagnosed with cancer X between enrollment in 1992 and June 30, 2007. Number of lifetime weight cycles was determined from questions on the baseline questionnaire asking how many times 10 or more pounds were intentionally lost and later regained.

Answer 3.29 Women with 10 + weight cycles have a higher BMI than other women, and BMI is "an established risk factor for cancer X." Therefore, adjustment for BMI would reduce the size of a positive association between having had 10 + weight cycles and cancer X.

Question 3.30 During 1987–2001, over 5000 persons ages 37–60 years with an elevated BMI ($\geq$ 34 for men, $\geq$ 38 for women) were recruited into a cohort study. A baseline physical exam was performed on each of them, and bariatric (weight loss) surgery was discussed. (The surgery entailed either restriction of the size of the stomach, its partial removal, or gastric bypass.) About 2000 cohort members opted for surgery, and the remaining participants formed the comparison ("non-exposed") group. All cohort members were monitored for fatal myocardial infarction through 2009.

The incidence of fatal heart attack in the persons who underwent bariatric surgery was 58% that in the nonexposed persons, and this was reduced further (to 52%) after adjustment for baseline characteristics, such as BMI, hypertension, and diabetes.

a. On the basis of the baseline characteristics (in aggregate) for which adjustment was performed, do you believe that persons in the surgery group were at the same, lower, or higher underlying risk of fatal myocardial infarction than persons in the nonsurgery group? Explain.

b. A skeptic of the results of this nonrandomized study argued that mismeasurement of some of these baseline characteristics led to an exaggerated estimate of benefit of bariatric surgery on the occurrence of fatal heart attack. Do you agree or disagree? Explain.

Answer 3.30

a. Because the adjusted estimate was lower than the crude relative risk, the surgery group must have been at an inherently greater risk of fatal MI than the nonsurgery group.

b. You disagree. The proposed misclassification of confounders in this study would have led to incomplete adjustment for confounding, causing the adjusted relative risk of 0.52 to be spuriously close to the crude relative risk of 0.58. More complete control of confounding would be expected to reduce the relative risk to a value below 0.52.

Question 3.31 A cohort study was conducted among pregnant women enrolled in the Medicaid program during 2000–2007. The prevalence of congenital malformations was compared between infants born to women who were (n = 1152) and were not (n = 885,844) taking a statin medication during the first trimester of pregnancy. Among statin users, 45.1% had a history of diabetes, compared with 3.1% of nonusers.

Among infants born to women who were statin users, the prevalence of a malformation (all types combined) was 6.34%, in contrast to 3.55% among other infants (relative risk = 1.79). After adjustment for the presence of maternal diabetes, the relative risk was 1.34.

From the above data, can you draw any conclusion as to the association of maternal diabetes and infant malformations in this study? If yes, what is it? If not, why not?

Answer 3.31 Women with diabetes were overrepresented among statin users. Only if maternal diabetes were itself associated with an increased risk of a congenital malformation could the relative risk adjusted for maternal diabetes turn out to be lower than the crude relative risk. Fetal exposure to statins was made to look relatively more harmful because such exposure tended to occur among diabetic women, women who already were at increased risk of delivering a malformed child.

(In this study, when further adjustment was done for age and other predictors of a malformation, there no longer was any association seen between statin use in pregnancy and risk of malformations.)

Question 3.32 Use of combined hormone therapy by post-menopausal women is associated with an increased incidence of breast cancer. Although the results of a randomized trial—the Women's Health Initiative (WHI)—suggest that breast cancer mortality also is increased among combined hormone users, results from nonrandomized studies suggest that there is no such increase. One possible explanation for the difference is the annual mammography screening that was provided to all participants in the randomized portion of the WHI study, whereas in the nonrandomized studies there likely was relatively greater receipt of screening mammography among women receiving hormones than among other women. Therefore, it is possible that the increased incidence seen among users of combined hormone therapy in the nonrandomized studies did not lead to a mortality increase because of the benefit achieved by the relatively high level of screening in these women.

If it were possible to ascertain receipt of screening mammography among women enrolled in the nonrandomized studies, would it be appropriate to adjust for this variable:

- to bring the results of these studies into better methodologic alignment with those from the WHI randomized trial?
- to estimate the influence of combined hormone therapy on breast cancer mortality among women in the population at large?

Answer 3.32 If the goal of the analysis were to estimate the impact of combined hormone therapy on breast cancer mortality, in the presence of a comparable level of screening mammography between treated and untreated women, then it would be appropriate to adjust for screening during the period of hormone use. However, probably of more practical value would be an analysis that examined the relationship without such an adjustment: if indeed hormone use leads to an increased level of screening, for many women the screening effectively becomes a part of the intervention, and should not be forced to be similar between hormone users and nonusers.

Question 3.33 Below are the results of a cohort study of American children that examined the occurrence of autism spectrum disorder (ASD) prior to age four years in relation to receipt of the first dose of MMR vaccine (typically administered between 12 and 15 months of age). Unlike most studies of this question, the present one had data on the occurrence of ASD in an older sibling, and stratified the data on this variable.

	Older Sibling without Autism Spectrum Disorder		Oldering Sibling with Autism Spectrum Disorder	
MMR status	Children with ASD	Total # of Children	Children with ASD	Total # of Children
Vaccinated	395	79,691	64	1491
Unvaccinated	65	11,957	25	387

a. Among children who were and were not vaccinated, respectively, what is the crude proportion who developed ASD by age four years?

b. Now adjusting for the ASD status of the older sibling, what is the proportion of unvaccinated children who developed ASD by age four years? (Use the distribution of ASD status in an older sibling of vaccinated children as the standard.)

c. What is the reason for the direction of the change from the crude incidence?

Answer 3.33

a. The crude cumulative incidence of ASD thru age four years:

Vaccinated: 459/81,182 = 5.65 per 1000
Unvaccinated: 90/12,344 = 7.29 per 1000

b. Among vaccinees, the proportion with a sibling without ASD was 79,691/(79,691 + 1491) = 0.982

The adjusted incidence of ASD in unvaccinated children would be

65/11,957 (0.982) + 25/387 (0.018) = 6.50 per 1000

c. The adjusted incidence among the unvaccinated is lower than the crude incidence of 7.29 per 1000. This is because the proportion of children with an older sibling with ASD—a factor associated with an increased risk of ASD in the younger sibling (see below)—was smaller among vaccinated children (the arbitrarily chosen reference population, 0.018) than among unvaccinated children (387/(11,957 + 387) = 0.031). Because the adjustment involved giving a relatively smaller weight to this high-risk stratum, the adjusted incidence among unvaccinated children was lower than the crude incidence. There is now less of a suggestion of a reduced risk of ASD in vaccinated children than when comparing the crude incidence figures.

[Among vaccinated children, the relative risk associated with having an older sibling with ASD was (64/1491)/(395/79,691) = 8.66. An elevation in risk also was present in unvaccinated children.]

CHAPTER **4**

Cohort Studies

COHORT STUDIES compare the occurrence of an illness or injury between persons with and without an exposure or characteristic. Threats to the validity of cohort studies can come from inaccurate characterization of exposure status; incomplete or inaccurate ascertainment of health outcomes; and differences between exposed and unexposed persons with respect to factors that themselves bear on the occurrence of the outcome. The forward-looking structure of cohort studies—start with exposure, follow subjects for the development of an outcome event—resembles that of randomized trials, and that similarity can put you off your guard when trying to interpret the results of such studies. The questions that follow are intended to put you back on guard.

Question 4.1 In a study of more than 20,000 women who had received a cosmetic breast implant (one that was not provided in relation to breast cancer surgery), all-cause mortality beginning 1 year later was only 74% that of socioeconomically and demographically comparable women in the population as a whole (95% CI = 0.68–0.81).[20] However, all-cause mortality in the implant recipients was nearly identical to that of some 16,000 women beginning 1 year after having undergone another form of cosmetic surgery during the same period of time (relative risk = 1.02, 95% CI = 0.89–1.17, adjusted for demographic characteristics).

Despite the observed 26% reduction in mortality compared to women in general, the authors concluded that the receipt of breast implants does not appear to influence death rates. Do you agree? If yes, why? If no, why not?

Answer 4.1 Women who have a serious illness are unlikely candidates for cosmetic implants; the proportion of women with such an illness is undoubtedly lower in the implant cohort than in the population as a whole (even after restricting the period of observation by excluding the first year after the operation). Thus, even in the absence of any influence of breast implants on the risk of death, the mortality experience of women receiving them would be expected to be more favorable than that of women in general. A better basis for comparison would be the death rates for the women undergoing other forms of cosmetic surgery, in which the same selection factors would be expected to be present. The similarity of death rates between implant recipients and other women undergoing cosmetic surgery argues that receipt of breast implants has no bearing on the risk of death.

Question 4.2 A study of the efficacy of pneumococcal vaccination in the elderly was described as follows[22]:

> We conducted a 2-year retrospective cohort study among all elderly members of a staff-model managed care organization who had a baseline diagnosis of chronic lung disease. The study outcomes were assessed over 2 years, from November 15, 1993, through November 14, 1995, and included hospitalizations for pneumonia and influenza.
>
> Of 1898 subjects, 1280 (67%) had received pneumococcal vaccination. This included 843 (44%) who were vaccinated prior to November 15, 1993 and an additional 437 (23%) vaccinated after that date. During the follow-up period there were 174 hospitalizations for pneumonia and influenza. The observed cumulative incidence was 138 per 1000 in the 618 unvaccinated persons and 70 per 1000 in the 1280 persons following their receipt of vaccination. This represents a 49% reduction in hospitalization for pneumonia and influenza.

Even if there were neither misclassification nor confounding in this study, the estimate of benefit associated with pneumococcal vaccination in elderly patients with chronic lung disease must be biased.

a. Why? In which direction?
b. How could the analysis be conducted to remove this source of bias?

Answer 4.2

a. Not all patients in this study were followed for the same length of time. Specifically, the 437 patients vaccinated during the 2-year study period were at risk for hospitalization only for the period after immunization. Thus, even had the hospitalization *rates* been the same in vaccinated and unvaccinated groups, the *cumulative incidence* would be lower in the former group. This would lead to an overestimate of the vaccine's efficacy.

b. The analysis should employ a person-time denominator, so that incidence rates can be calculated. The 437 persons vaccinated after November 15, 1993, would contribute person-time-at-risk to the experience of the *un*vaccinated persons until their date of vaccination, and to the experience of vaccinated persons afterward. Because the risk of hospitalization for pneumonia and influenza may be relatively low in the several week period immediately after November 15 (i.e., before the seasonal peak), adjustment for calendar period may be needed. Otherwise, confounding could arise from the different calendar distribution of person-time between vaccinated and unvaccinated groups.

Question 4.3 The following is taken from the abstract of an article on the mortality experience of employees at a polymer manufacturing facility, the DuPont Washington Works plant in West Virginia[23]:

> *Methods.* The cohort comprised 6,027 men and women who had worked at the facility between 1948 and 2002; these years delimit the mortality follow-up period. Standardized mortality ratios (SMRs) were estimated to compare the observed number of deaths to expected numbers derived from mortality rates for 2 reference populations: the West Virginia state population and an 8-state regional employee population from the same company.

The results of the study for deaths from heart disease are shown in the table below. (The SMRs presented are adjusted for age, sex, and calendar time.)

SMR estimates with 95% confidence intervals for mortality for heart disease for all Washington Works employees compared to 2 external reference populations

Cause of death	WW cohort O	WV population E	SMR	95% CI	DuPont 8-state regional employee population E	SMR	95% CI
All heart disease	314	475.6	66.0	58.9, 73.7	284.5	110.4	98.5, 123.3

WW = Washington Works; WV = West Virginia; O = observed deaths; E = expected deaths; SMR = standardized mortality ratio = O/E x 100%; CI = confidence interval.

The confidence intervals around the SMRs based on expected deaths in the DuPont Region 1 workers are somewhat wider than those based on expected deaths in West Virginia. Nonetheless, when evaluating the possible impact of employment at the Washington Works plant on mortality from heart disease, why might the SMRs based on death rates in DuPont Region 1 workers provide a more valid estimate?

Answer 4.3 Persons with heart disease are less likely than other persons to become employed and stay employed, and also are more likely to die of heart disease. The proportion of WW employees with heart disease is almost certainly smaller than in the West Virginia population, leading to a spuriously low estimate of relative mortality from heart disease when these population death rates are used as a basis for comparison. A similar distortion would not be expected to be present using mortality rates of other workers as a means of determining the expected number of deaths.

Question 4.4 In Paris in the 1830s, bloodletting was believed to be efficacious in the treatment of pneumonia (and a number of other diseases). Virtually all patients diagnosed with pneumonia underwent this treatment, some early in the course of the disease and some later. Louis compared the case-fatality in 41 patients with pneumonia who were bled within the first 4 days of disease onset with that in 36 others who were bled later. The number of deaths were 18 and 9 in the two groups (case-fatality = 44% and 25%, respectively). While the early-bled cases were somewhat older than the late-bled cases (41 vs. 38 years), Louis concluded that "the effect of venesection [i.e., blood letting] on the progress of pneumonitis is much less than is commonly thought."

Presented with these data, today's epidemiologists would exclude from the analysis the experience during the first 4 days following disease onset, and would not calculate case-fatality from disease onset but rather mortality rates starting on day 5 (for the early-bled groups) or from the time bloodletting began (late-bled group), adjusting for number of days since disease onset. What would be the rationale for this modified approach? Do you expect that today's method would raise or lower the estimate of relative risk of death associated with receiving early blood letting?

Answer 4.4 A comparison of case-fatality from the time of disease onset inflates the relative case-fatality associated with early bleeding, given that deaths that occur during the 4 days following disease onset can be only in the early-bled group. The rate-based approach that takes this into account, and also adjusts for time since disease onset (after four days), will produce a relative risk of death associated with early blood letting that is lower—as long as some deaths do occur within the first four days after illness onset.

Question 4.5 This question is based on the following abstract (abridged):

Methods We conducted a retrospective cohort study of post-war mortality according to cause among 695,516 Gulf War veterans and 746,291 other veterans. The follow-up continued through September 1993. A stratified, multivariate analysis (with Cox proportional-hazards models) controlled for branch of service, type of unit, age, sex, and race in comparing the two groups. We used standardized mortality ratios to compare the groups of veterans with the general population of the United States.

Results Among the Gulf War veterans, there was a small but significant excess of deaths as compared with the veterans who did not serve in the Persian Gulf (adjusted rate ratio, 1.09; 95 percent confidence interval, 1.01 to 1.16). In both groups of veterans the mortality rates were lower overall than those in the general population. The adjusted standardized mortality ratios were 0.44 (95 percent confidence interval, 0.42 to 0.47) for Gulf War veterans and 0.38 (0.36 to 0.40) for other veterans.

(N ENGL J MED 1996;335:1498-504.)

The veterans who served in the Persian Gulf War had a postwar mortality that was 9% higher than that of other veterans, but only 44% that of Americans in general. Which of these figures do you believe is most likely to reflect the subsequent impact (if any) of having experienced the Persian Gulf War? Why?

Answer 4.5 A comparison of mortality in Gulf War veterans to that in similar-aged Americans in general would likely be biased, since persons with a number of diseases would not be eligible for military service and would also be at an increased risk of death during 1991–1993. The more appropriate comparison group is that of veterans who did not serve in the Persian Gulf (which produced the rate ratio of 1.09).

Question 4.6 A cohort study was conducted among 6,849 Swedish men with localized prostate cancer diagnosed during 1997–2002.[24] Death rates through 2008 were compared between those who did and did not undergo treatment with curative intent (most commonly, a radical prostatectomy). The cumulative 10-year mortality from prostate cancer was low (2.7 per 100) in the men receiving an attempt at cure, and only 0.9 per 100 higher than this in those not so treated. About 10 per 100 of the actively treated men died of causes other than prostate cancer; adjusting for age, the corresponding figure for the men in whom a curative procedure was not attempted was nearly twice as high.

The very large observed difference in mortality from causes other than prostate cancer was almost certainly not the result of chance, and it seems unlikely to be a result of an attempt to cure localized prostate cancer. What do you believe to be the explanation?

Answer 4.6 When interpreting the results of any cohort study, it is always necessary to ask, "Could some reason for the presence or level of exposure itself bear a relation to the outcome in question?" In this instance, it seems likely that one factor entering into the decision to attempt a curative procedure in a man with localized prostate cancer is the perceived life expectancy of that man: The presence of a life-shortening condition (e.g., heart disease, some other form of cancer) would argue against an intervention that (even though potentially curative) would entail its own morbidity. As a result of this source of confounding, the observed reduction in mortality from causes other than prostate cancer associated with active treatment almost certainly does not reflect a benefit of that treatment.

Question 4.7 This question is based on an excerpt of an abstract of a published article[25]:

Background. Reports on the relation between anthropometric variables (height, weight) and physical activity with ovarian cancer have been inconclusive. The objective of the current study was to extend investigation of potential associations in the Iowa Women's Health Study cohort.

Methods. The relation between self-reported anthropometric variables and incident ovarian cancer was studied in a prospective cohort of women ages 55–69 years who were followed for 15 years. Two hundred twenty-three incident cases of epithelial ovarian cancer were identified by linkage to a cancer registry.

Results. No association was found overall between ovarian cancer and height. Although current body mass index (BMI) was not associated with ovarian cancer, a BMI ≥30 kg/m2 at age 18 years appeared to be associated positively with ovarian cancer (multivariate-adjusted RR, 1.83 for BMI ≥30 kg/m2 vs. BMI <25 kg/m2; 95% CI, 0.90–3.72), and this association was stronger after exclusion of the first 2 years of follow-up (RR, 2.15; 95% CI, 1.05–4.40).

Conclusions. Anthropometric variables were not major risk factors for ovarian cancer in the cohort studied; however, high BMI in early adulthood may increase the risk of ovarian cancer among postmenopausal women.

In some cohort studies, events and person-time in exposed and unexposed persons begins only after a period of time has elapsed following formation of the cohort. When evaluating the possible influence of BMI at age 18 years as a predictor of risk of ovarian cancer in the Iowa Women's Health Study, would you recommend that approach, or instead one in which events and person-time are tabulated right away? Why?

Answer 4.7 The exclusion of events for a period of time following the formation of a cohort is appropriate if there is concern that there are occult cases of disease among cohort members in whom exposure status ascertained at the beginning of follow-up does not reflect that at the time their disease was being produced. For the variable BMI at age 18, this is of no concern, given that the earliest a woman's follow-up could begin was at age 55. The appropriate analysis in this study should consider events and person-time from the very start of follow-up.

Question 4.8 A British study enrolled a large number of post-menopausal women attending a breast cancer screening program and ascertained whether they were or were not taking hormone replacement therapy (HRT) at that time.[26] During the follow-up period, 2,894 users of HRT at baseline developed breast cancer, versus 3,202 never users, producing a relative risk of 1.66. Deaths from breast cancer occurred in 238 users of HRT at baseline and in 191 never users (relative risk = 1.22).

A letter to the editor (*Lancet* 2003;362:329) argued that

> the data provided for breast-cancer mortality are somewhat misleading. Compared with never-users of HRT the relative risk of death from breast cancer was raised in current-users. However, this finding should not be interpreted as evidence that HRT increases the risk of mortality among women diagnosed with breast cancer; the overall breast-cancer mortality rate will necessarily be higher in current-users as a result of the higher frequency of breast cancer among such women. To quote breast-cancer mortality figures for the subgroup of women diagnosed with breast cancer would seem more appropriate—i.e., never-users of HRT, mortality rate 8.2% (238 of 2894) versus current-users of HRT, mortality rate 6.0% (191 of 3202). These figures give a crude relative risk estimate of 0.725 for current-users versus never-users for breast-cancer mortality, indicating a lower risk of death in women taking HRT at the time of their diagnosis with breast cancer than in never-users.

Which of the two approaches to gauging mortality from breast cancer in women who use HRT—that of the authors of the study, or that of the authors of the letter to the editor—has the potential to provide data that are "somewhat misleading"? Why?

Answer 4.8 The data produced by the authors of the letter are misleading. A comparison of the risk of death from breast cancer in women who do and do not receive HRT needs to incorporate the possible influence of HRT on both incidence and on case-fatality. The use of mortality rates in users and nonusers by the authors of the article does this; the use of case-fatality alone does not.

Question 4.9 A meta-analysis of 13 studies of mortality from brain cancer among firefighters obtained a summary standardized mortality ratio (SMR) of 1.09 (95% CI = 0.92–1.25).[27] Using data from six of these studies that provided results based on duration of employment, a second meta-analysis conducted by the same author showed the following:

Duration of employment (years)	Observed	Expected	SMR
<10	8	6.50	1.23
10–19	12	7.41	1.62
20–29	11	6.30	1.75
≥30	11	5.24	2.10

Put aside the possible concern with "healthy worker" or other form of bias in these studies. Also, assume that both duration of firefighting employment and death from brain cancer have been ascertained without error. Explain why the SMRs above likely overstate the association between any particular duration of firefighting and mortality from brain cancer.

Answer 4.9 A weighted average of the SMRs in the table would give an overall SMR considerably greater than the value of 1.09 that is based on the results of all studies. The results of the six studies are not representative of the entire group of 13, most likely as a result of a form of publication bias—the tendency of authors reporting the results of individual studies to preferentially present positive results. Plausibly, the authors of one or more of the remaining seven studies examined SMRs by duration of employment, obtained a null or inverse relation, and chose to provide to readers only the data for all durations combined.

Question 4.10 In a randomized controlled trial of screening for two forms of cancer (breast and colon), more than 150,000 men and women were recruited to take part. Follow-up of these individuals took place over an average of 5 years for cancer incidence and cause-specific mortality.

In an analysis unrelated to those bearing on the efficacy of screening, incidence and mortality rates in all trial participants combined were compared to those of demographically comparable individuals in the population as a whole. The incidence of cancer (excluding cancer of the breast and colon) in the trial participants was 89% that of the general population, whereas the corresponding figure for cancer mortality was 56%.

Because of the large number of events, chance is a highly unlikely explanation for the difference between the relative risk for cancer incidence (0.89) and that for cancer mortality (0.56). What do you believe to be the most likely explanation for the difference?

Answer 4.10 Persons dying of cancer are unlikely to be participants in a cancer screening program. Their exclusion from the study participants, but not from the comparison population, would be expected to have a large impact on relative cancer mortality but little or none on relative cancer incidence. This represents a form of "healthy screenee bias."[28]

Question 4.11 The occurrence of transient neurologic symptoms (transient ischemic attacks, TIA) commonly heralds the later occurrence of a stroke (with its associated nontransient neurologic damage). In 1,707 patients with a TIA, a stroke took place in the subsequent 90 days in 14% of the 235 who received warfarin anticoagulation therapy at the time of the TIA and in 10% of the other TIA patients (p = .04). The latter patients generally received aspirin or no specific therapy.

The authors of this study warned that despite the excellent quality of information on treatment received and on outcome events, the study may not provide valid data on the (lack of) efficacy of warfarin anticoagulation in persons with a TIA. What do you believe is the primary basis for their cautious interpretation?

Answer 4.11 The authors likely are concerned with the presence of confounding—among patients with a TIA, warfarin anticoagulation treatment may have been selectively administered to those with an inherently greater stroke risk (perhaps based on age or the severity of the transient episode).

Question 4.12 Investigators at a clinic specializing in post-trauma care wished to determine whether persons who sustain acute neck trauma are at an increased risk of developing a diffuse pain syndrome (i.e., involving multiple parts of the body). They identified 102 patients in their clinic an average of 12 months after neck trauma, in whom 22 (21.6%) had symptoms that met the criteria for diffuse pain syndrome (DPS). In contrast, among 59 patients seen in the clinic an average of 12 months after a lower extremity fracture, only 1 (1.7%) reported symptoms consistent with DPS ($p = 0.001$). Based in large part on the strong association observed in this study, a review article concluded that the hypothesis that acute neck trauma can trigger DPS "meets established criteria for determining causality."

In this study, not all patients who sustained a neck injury were included, but rather just those who sought care in the clinic. Under what circumstance could this choice have led to a spurious exaggeration of the association between neck injury and DPS? (Assume that demographic and other risk factors for DPA are comparable between the patients with neck injury and those with lower extremity fracture.)

Answer 4.12 It may be that most or all patients with a lower extremity fracture require continuing care through 12 months postfracture, in other words, they will be seen even in the absence of any new condition. If the same were not true for neck trauma patients, then those seeking care from the clinic an average of 12 months later will be over-represented by patients with new problems, including DPS. Only a cohort study that monitors the later DPS status of *all* victims of neck and lower extremity trauma can be trusted to provide a valid result.

Question 4.13 You are planning a cohort study of the possible influence of elective induction of labor at 39 weeks' gestation on the risk of several adverse maternal and fetal outcomes, including the need for cesarean section. As a basis for comparison to the women receiving elective induction, you are considering two possibilities:

(a) Women who delivered a child at 39 weeks who went into labor spontaneously and (like the women who were electively induced) did not have any indication for induction (e.g., preeclampsia, gestational diabetes)

(b) Women who at 39 weeks had not yet delivered and (as of that time) had no indication for induction.

Which of (a) or (b) would be the more likely to provide an unbiased estimate?

Answer 4.13 The correct answer is (b), because in this clinical scenario the alternative to a decision to electively induce labor at 39 weeks is to allow the pregnancy to continue. While some women whose delivery is not induced will indeed soon deliver on their own, others will remain pregnant at 40 weeks and beyond, during which time pregnancy complications often develop. These complications may lead to the decision to induce labor for medical reasons or to perform a cesarean section. Women experiencing these outcomes would be inappropriately excluded from comparison group (a). All of the women not undergoing elective induction of labor must be retained in the comparison population so as to obtain a valid assessment of the experience associated with this alternative course of action.

This has been noted by Caughey et al.,[29] who also provided some illustrative data on the occurrence of cesarean section:

Induction of labor at 39 weeks?*	% of women delivered by cesarean section
Yes	14.3%
No	
Delivered at 39 weeks	9.1%
Delivered after 39 weeks	15.0%

*These generally were not elective inductions, but the presence of an indication for induction was adjusted for in the analysis.

The use of noninduced women who delivered at 39 weeks as a basis for the expected incidence of cesarean section would incorrectly suggest that induction of labor at 39 weeks predisposed to this outcome.

The didactic message: Comparison groups in cohort studies should not be subject to selection on the basis of events that occur after the time that the exposure has been sustained.

Question 4.14 The following questions pertain to a table from a British cohort study of lung cancer mortality in relation to occupational asbestos exposure and cigarette smoking.

Smoking Status	Asbestos Exposure	Deaths	Person-years	RR	(95% CI)
Never	Low	8	280 812	1.0	—
	Medium	19	127 484	1.9	(0.8–4.3)
	High	8	23 686	1.6	(0.6–4.2)
Former	Low	61	156 892	5.6	(2.7–11.7)
	Medium	125	143 494	6.5	(3.2–13.3)
	High	116	48 028	9.7	(4.7–20.0)
Current	Low	473	581 497	18.8	(9.4–37.9)
	Medium	636	257 181	22.7	(11.3–45.6)
	High	322	50 590	26.2	(13.0–53.1)

Relative risk (RR) adjusted for age, calendar period, and sex; " Low," < 10 years occupational exposure to asbestos; "Medium," 10–29 years occupational exposure to asbestos; "High," ≥ 30 years occupational exposure to asbestos.

(a) In their description of the study methods, the authors stated that person-years were calculated from the date of first employment in an industry in which asbestos exposure was likely to have taken place. If person-years had, in fact, been tabulated in this manner, a strong bias would have been present. Why? In which direction?

(b) Inspection of the data in the table suggests that, in fact, persons in the "Medium" and "High" categories of asbestos exposure did *not* accrue person-years from the time of first employment. Why is this?

Answer 4.14

(a) This is an example of "immortal time" bias. Among persons with ≥ 30 years of occupational exposure to asbestos, no deaths could have occurred within the first 29 years. Among persons with 10–29 years of occupational exposure, no deaths could have occurred in the first nine years. No such person-time free of risk is present in the group with "Low" (< 10 years) exposure. This inflation of the denominator of the "High" and "Medium" groups would lead to death rates in them that would be spuriously low.

   Person-time in the "High" and "Medium" groups should begin to accrue only after the duration criterion for eligibility is met (at 30 years and 10 years, respectively).

(b) Because the number of person-years used in calculating mortality rates is smaller in the "High" and "Medium" groups than in the "Low" group, it is clear that person-years were not accrued from first employment, but rather from the time that the duration criterion was met.

Question 4.15 The following is adapted from the abstract of an article:

Since 1973 we have identified and longitudinally followed 73 asymptomatic, apparently healthy subjects with frequent and complex ventricular ectopy. . . . Subjects came to medical attention because of the accidental or incidental discovery of frequent and complex ventricular ectopy through standard electrocardiography or routine physical examination and were subsequently referred for cardiologic evaluation. Subjects gave a complete medical history and underwent physical examination. . . . The consistency of the frequent and complex ventricular ectopy was confirmed by . . . electrocardiographic re-examination. Subjects in whom any cardiac disease was indicated by any noninvasive diagnostic test were excluded from the study. Subjects documented to have no detectable cardiac disease were entered into the longitudinal follow-up study.

Follow-up for 3.0 to 9.5 years (mean, 6.5) was accomplished in 70 subjects (96%) and documented one sudden death and one death from cancer. Calculation of a standardized mortality ratio (U.S. data, 8th revision) for 448 person-years of follow-up indicated that 7.4 deaths were expected, whereas 2 occurred. . . . We conclude that the long-term prognosis in otherwise healthy subjects with frequent and complex ventricular ectopy is similar to or better than that of members of the U.S. population at large.

The standardized mortality ratio referred to above effectively controlled for possible confounding by age, sex, race, and time period. Nonetheless, you are concerned that the authors' concluding sentence might be too optimistic. Why?

Answer 4.15 The 73 members of the cohort with complex ventricular ectopy were drawn from a larger group that had undergone noninvasive diagnostic testing for the presence of cardiac disease. Those persons with evidence of cardiac disease were excluded. No similar restriction was placed on the comparison "group," that is, death rates in the U.S. population. This incomparability would be expected to lead to a substantial degree of "healthy screenee" bias, distorting the comparison and resulting in a spuriously low relative risk of death in persons with complex ventricular ectopy.

Question 4.16 In a cohort study, women who had undergone apparently successful treatment of advanced ovarian cancer later received additional surgery to identify and attempt to remove any remaining malignancy. Among the women, those who had no tumor or very little tumor remaining after such "second look" surgery had a much better prognosis than those with a considerable amount of residual tumor. However, a randomized trial of "second look" surgery observed no difference in survival between women assigned to the surgical arm and women not offered additional surgery.

Assume that both studies were very large and otherwise well done. What do you believe is the likeliest explanation for the association seen in the cohort study?

Answer 4.16 There was undoubtedly a great deal of confounding in the cohort study. Women with less widespread disease (and thus an inherently better prognosis) would be expected to have less residual tumor after the second surgery than women with more widespread disease. Based on the results of the randomized trial, the surgery appears to have contributed little or nothing to the survival in these women.

Question 4.17 Children born with cardiac malformation X are cyanotic, and they typically undergo cardiac surgery during the first several days of life. Those who survive the operation generally are discharged from the hospital after three to four weeks.

You have the ability to identify all infants with malformation X who were discharged alive in the state of Washington during 2013, and wish to determine whether they are subject to excess mortality during the remainder of the first year of life. You plan to enumerate deaths among members of this cohort and to compare their cumulative mortality to that of newborns in the state of Washington thru 12 months of age. The comparison group's infant mortality can be obtained from data routinely generated by the Vital Records division of Washington State.

Assume complete ascertainment of mortality, and that the condition is rare enough so that there is no appreciable bias resulting from the inclusion of the infants with malformation X in the comparison group. What do you believe to be the greatest threat to the validity of the planned research approach? Why? Would the results over- or under-estimate the relative mortality of infants with malformation X who were discharged alive after cardiac surgery?

Answer 4.17 Infants in the comparison group are at risk of dying during the first three to four weeks of life, whereas by definition infants in the malformation X cohort have survived this period of time. As a result of this "immortal time" bias, the malformation X cohort members will appear to have a falsely favorable relative survival.

Question 4.18 Interviews were conducted with 49 children (and/or their parents) with current evidence of impairment of renal function. Of the nine children who previously had undergone renal transplantation, six (67%) met the criteria for depression, in contrast to only seven of 40 children (17.5%) who had not met the criteria (p < .05). What aspect of the design of this study is of particular concern when seeking to infer whether, among children with renal disease, receipt of a transplant is a risk factor for depression later in childhood?

Answer 4.18 The higher prevalence of depression among children who had received a renal transplant and have *current* evidence of impaired renal function is likely quite different than that among pediatric transplant recipients in general (many of whom no longer have impaired renal function). It could easily be true that it is not the transplant per se, but rather the at-least-partial failure of the transplant that is giving rise to depression.

Question 4.19 A cohort study of the efficacy of traditional Chinese medicine (TCM) in the treatment of advanced breast cancer was conducted. The investigators identified 729 women who were diagnosed with breast cancer during 2001–2010 and who went on to receive taxane treatment (which would be given only for the presence of advanced disease). Among these women, 115 received TCM for at least one month before and/or after the initial administration of taxane treatment. Survival from the index date (the date on which taxane treatment was initiated) was compared between the women who did and did not receive TCM, and was greater in the former group. The survival advantage among users of TCM was particularly great in those women who received TCM for more than six months.

Assume that the difference in survival between TCM users and nonusers was not the result of chance, and was not due to confounding (i.e., an inherently better prognosis in TCM users). Nonetheless, it is likely that the observed association is due wholly or in part to a distortion resulting from the study's design and analysis. What is the nature of that distortion? Why would it lead to a spuriously large survival difference between women treated with TCM and other women with advanced breast cancer?

Answer 4.19 In this study, survival among women who initiated treatment with TCM after taxane use had begun should have been measured NOT from the start of treatment with a taxane, but from the date that a patient had completed one month of use of TCM (six months for women in the category of users for 6 + months). Survival among women with advanced breast cancer who were not treated with TCM should be measured beginning at the corresponding times following their own diagnoses.

Measuring survival from the index date (start of treatment with a taxane) allowed women who later went on to receive TCM to have been "immortal" for that period of time between the index date and the completion of one month of TCM, leading to an apparent improvement in survival even if TCM had no actual impact on prognosis.

Question 4.20 A group of investigators reported on the survival of women treated for breast cancer at their institution from 1935 to 1982:

Over the period of the study, no significant change was noted in overall survival. However, survival among patients with metastatic disease at the time of diagnosis of breast cancer improved substantially. The median age-adjusted survival of such patients in the period 1934–1954 was six months; in the period 1955–1974 it increased to 21 months; and in the period 1975–1982 it increased further to 28 months. This increased survival is probably related to advances in therapy, such as combination chemotherapy.

Apart from chance, what is yet another explanation for the findings regarding the change over time in survival among women with metastatic disease?

Answer 4.20 If the means of identifying the presence of metastatic disease had improved (and/or were more commonly used) between 1934 and 1954 and between 1975 and 1982, the true increase in survival over time would have been overestimated. The additional patients diagnosed as having metastatic disease in the later time period would likely have had less advanced cancer, on average, than the patients who would have been diagnosed using just the earlier technology. This would have resulted in a difference in the underlying life expectancy in the groups of women diagnosed as having "metastatic" disease during the different periods of time. In turn, this would have led to an increase in measured survival over time among women labeled as having "metastatic" breast cancer, even in the absence of any differences in the efficacy of treatment.

Question 4.21 The following question pertains to an abridged Abstract of an article, "Aspirin and mortality from coronary bypass surgery."

ABSTRACT

Background: Because platelet activation constitutes a pivotal mechanism for injury in patients with atherosclerosis, we assessed whether early treatment with aspirin could improve survival after coronary bypass surgery.

Methods: At 70 centers in 17 countries, we prospectively studied 5065 patients undergoing coronary bypass surgery, of whom 5022 survived the first 48 hours after surgery.

Results: Among patients who received aspirin (up to 650 mg) within 48 hours after revascularization, subsequent mortality was 1.3% (40 of 2999 patients), as compared with 4.0% among those who did not receive aspirin during this period (81 of 2023, P < 0.001). Aspirin therapy was associated with a 48% reduction in the incidence of myocardial infarction (2.8% vs. 5.4%, P < 0.001), a 50% reduction in the incidence of stroke (1.3% vs. 2.6%, P = 0.01), a 74% reduction in the incidence of renal failure (0.9% vs. 3.4%, P < 0.001), and a 62% reduction in the incidence of bowel infarction (0.3% vs. 0.8, P = 0.01):

Conclusion: Early use of aspirin after coronary bypass surgery is associated with a reduced risk of death and ischemic complications involving the heart, brain, kidneys, and gastrointestinal tract.

N Engl J Med 2002; 347: 1309–17

An accompanying editorial stated that this "report might actually underestimate the benefit of early aspirin use (since) the deaths that occurred in the first 48 hours after coronary bypass surgery were not included in the analysis." Those deaths occurred in 41 of 2064 patients not receiving aspirin during the first 48 hours and in only two of 3001 patients who did. You believe that in the analysis of mortality, inclusion of deaths that occurred in the first 48 hours after surgery actually would lead to a spuriously large estimate of the beneficial influence of aspirin treatment that was administered during those 48 hours. Why?

Answer 4.21 Patients who received aspirin in the first 48 hours after surgery must have survived long enough to have been given this medication. No such "guarantee" of survival during the early postoperative period would be present among patients who did not receive aspirin. The "immortal time" bias that would be manifest in an analysis that included the period of time beginning immediately following surgery would lead to a result that would suggest a falsely large mortality benefit associated with aspirin treatment. The bias can be prevented by doing exactly what was done by the authors of the study: beginning follow-up in aspirin-treated and other patients once the period for determining exposure status has concluded, that is, as of 48 hours post-surgery.

Question 4.22 From a national surveillance program in England and Wales for the years 2009–2012, investigators identified 75 pregnant women who sustained a laboratory-confirmed invasive Hemophilus influenza infection.[31] These cases were diagnosed in all three trimesters; the median gestational age at the time of diagnosis was 20 weeks.

Fetal loss occurred in 47 of these pregnancies (61%). From existing data, the investigators estimated that 21% of pregnancies in general among British women resulted in fetal loss, and, therefore, that the relative risk of fetal loss associated with invasive H influenza infection was 2.9.

The relative risk of 2.9 associated with invasive H influenza infection that was obtained in this analysis is likely to be a considerable underestimate of the true relative risk. Why?

Answer 4.22 Many fetal losses occur early in pregnancy. The appropriate means of gauging the potential impact of an invasive H influenza infection on pregnancy loss is to compare the experience of women with such an infection with that of uninfected women who have the identical distribution of durations of pregnancy as the "exposed" cohort.

The median gestational age at the time of infection was 20 weeks. Therefore, the percentage of comparison women who went on to sustain a fetal loss during that part of pregnancy in which the infected women were at risk of a loss would have to be considerably lower than 21% (the figure pertaining to losses counted from the time of conception), and so the true relative risk would have to be larger than 2.9.

Question 4.23 In 1991, the state of California began to prohibit the purchase of a handgun by persons who had been convicted of a violent misdemeanor in the prior 10 years. To evaluate the impact of this law, investigators identified 927 persons under 35 years of age who in 1991 were denied permission to purchase a handgun on this basis. The rate of arrest for violent crimes by these persons during the next three years was compared to that of 727 persons under 35 years of age who purchased handguns in 1989–1990 but who, had the law been in effect at the time, would similarly have been denied. The cumulative incidence of arrest for a violent crime was 29% higher in the 1989–1990 cohort than in the 1991 cohort.

Assume that there were no differences in demographic characteristics between the two cohorts. What further assumption is needed for the observed difference of 29% to be judged as truly reflecting the impact of the legislation?

Answer 4.23 It is necessary to assume that the other determinants of violent crime by persons with a history of a violent misdemeanor did not differ between the two cohorts (i.e., had not been changing over time). The authors noted that during the period of the study, the incidence of violent crime in general had increased somewhat. This suggests that, if anything, the observed relative risk of 1.29 could be a modest underestimate of the true impact of the law.

Question 4.24 Stillbirths are defined as fetal deaths occurring in pregnancies of 20 weeks duration or longer. Gestational diabetes is defined as diabetes that is first diagnosed during pregnancy. The large majority of cases of gestational diabetes are diagnosed by means of blood glucose screening during the 24th–28th weeks of pregnancy.

The following data regarding stillbirth occurrence in relation to gestational diabetes were obtained from a study conducted in a large population. (Women diagnosed with diabetes prior to the pregnancy have been excluded.)

Gestational Diabetes	Number of Stillbirths	Number of Pregnancies	Risk of Stillbirth per 1,000
Yes	323	76,669	4.2
No	9,165	1,925,080	4.8

The comparison of the risk of stillbirth between women with and without gestational diabetes is biased.

a. Why, and in which direction?
b. Assuming data are available on gestational age at the time of the stillbirth, how could the data be analyzed to remove the bias?

Answer 4.24

(a) The presence of gestational diabetes generally was not ascertained until at least week 24, so fetal deaths between weeks 20 and 24 could occur only among women without gestational diabetes (or women not known to have it at the time the fetal death occurred). This would generate a spuriously low relative incidence of stillbirths in women with gestational diabetes.

(b) The bias can be eliminated by tabulating stillbirth occurrence in all women starting in the 29th week of pregnancy, that is, *after* all of them have been evaluated for the presence of gestational diabetes.

CHAPTER 5

Case-Control Studies

IN CASE-CONTROL STUDIES, persons with a given illness or injury (cases) are characterized as to whether or not they previously had sustained a given exposure (and degree of that exposure). Ideally, as a basis for comparison, we would like to determine the probability and degree of exposure in a sample of a population from which the cases were drawn. This ideal can be hard to achieve in practice, and it is common for the results of case-control studies to be ambiguous in their interpretation. Nonetheless, because case-control studies potentially are able to provide valid results, and because there are instances in which the only data relevant to a particular etiologic relation can be obtained from case-control studies, they are, warts and all, an essential item in the epidemiologist's toolbox.

Question 5.1 The following is excerpted from a letter to the editor of a medical journal:

> The fact that several relatives sometimes stutter has led others to assert that stuttering is inherited. Yet in forty years of experience I have met more stutterers who had no close relatives or ancestors who stuttered than those who had. It is my observation that most stutterers are hypersensitive persons, and I believe that hypersensitivity is acquired at an early age through the child's environment.

Does the information in the letter address the possible association between positive family history of stuttering and stuttering itself? If yes, how? If no, why not?

Answer 5.1 Even though only a minority of stutterers have a family history of this condition, that proportion may still be considerably in excess of the proportion present among nonstutterers. In the absence of data on the latter, no conclusions can be drawn regarding the presence or absence of an association.

Question 5.2 In a case-control study of pneumonia in infants in southern Brazil, the mothers of 152 cases and 2,391 controls were interviewed. A far higher proportion of cases than controls were not being breast-fed during the week prior to the date of onset of the case's illness (and the corresponding date for controls): odds ratio = 17, 95% confidence interval = 7.7–36.0.

A commentator on this study indicated that a "serious concern is the relatively small sample size, with the result that very few cases were exclusively breast fed." Do you agree that this is a "serious concern" when interpreting the results of the study? If yes, why? If no, why not?

Answer 5.2 No. The lower confidence limit of the odds ratio associated with not breast-feeding is 7.7; thus, there is little possibility that chance is solely responsible for the association. There would be concern over the sample size only if it were important to know more precisely where, within the range of 7.7–36.0, the true odds ratio lies.

Question 5.3 You are planning to conduct a case-control study that would examine a possible association between a genetic characteristic—called T1—and the incidence of lung cancer. About 10% of the population possesses T1. In this study, you have two laboratory methods that potentially could be used to measure a person's T1 status from a sample of his/her DNA. Neither is perfect. Method A will correctly categorize everyone who truly is positive for T1, but is expected to misclassify 5% of truly negative persons as being T1-positive. Conversely, method B will correctly classify everyone who is truly T1-negative, but will misclassify 5% of T1-positive persons as T1-negative. Which is the better choice of tests to minimize bias in the odds ratio relating T1 status and lung cancer?

a. Method A
b. Method B
c. Neither is a better choice than the other.

Explain your answer.

Answer 5.3 Method B will provide a less biased result, since its use will result in a relatively smaller proportion of misclassified individuals. As an example:

True T1 status	Cases	Controls	Odds Ratio
+	200	100	2.25
−	800	900	

Using Method A, 5% × 800 = 40 cases truly negative for T1 would be labeled as T1–positive, as would 5% × 900 = 45 controls.

Method A: Observed T1 status	Cases	Controls	
+	200 + 40	100 + 45	1.64
−	800 − 40	900 − 45	

Using Method B, 5% × 200 = 10 cases truly positive for T1 would be labeled as T1-negative, as would 5% × 100 = 5 controls.

Method B: Observed T1 status	Cases	Controls	
+	200 − 10	100 − 5	1.99
−	800 + 10	800 + 5	

Question 5.4 The following is excerpted from an article on potential risks associated with spray painting in the automobile industry[30]:

> In the case-control analyses, cases are defined as all lung cancer deaths among the automotive workers (n = 263). Controls are defined as those deaths due to circulatory disease or to accidents among those same workers, thus ensuring a valid representation of the population under investigation.

In this study, a history of spray painting was ascertained in cases and controls from company records.

a. What "population" is the one for which we would like to know the proportion of employees who worked as spray painters?
b. Apart from chance, how might the control group selected not accurately characterize the proportion exposed in that population?

Answer 5.4

a. The population is that of automotive workers at risk of death in the period during which case accrual took place.

b. If work as a spray painter is associated with the rate of death of the two causes selected—positively or negatively—then the proportion of spray painters in this control group will not be representative of that in the underlying population at risk.

Question 5.5 At the sexually transmitted infection (STI) clinic where you work, you are planning a case-control study of acute gonorrhea in men in relation to condom use. Because the cases of gonorrhea seen at the clinic are not derived from any defined population, you consider the use of male patients with an STI other than gonorrhea as a sampling frame for controls. This choice has the advantage of being feasible, and it is likely that the accuracy of information obtained on recent condom use would be similar between cases and controls. What do you believe to be the primary threat to the validity of this study if you were to select as controls men seen at the clinic for an STI other than gonorrhea?

Answer 5.5 The primary concern here is selection bias. Condom use (or the lack thereof) plausibly has a similar favorable impact on the incidence of both gonorrhea and other STIs. Therefore, the prevalence of condom use in STI controls may be considerably lower than in men in general. The use of such a control group could lead to a spuriously low estimate of the efficacy of condom use in the prevention of gonorrhea.

Question 5.6 This question is based on the following abstract.[32]

Study objective. To investigate the association of alcohol use and night driving with traumatic snowmobile fatalities.

Design. Case-control study.

Participants. Traumatic deaths occurring while driving a snowmobile during the years 1985 to 1990 were reviewed. A sample of 1989 to 1990 fatal motor vehicle driver and motorcycle driver accidents were used as controls. Records were obtained from the provincial coroner.

Results. One hundred eight snowmobile fatalities, 432 motor vehicle fatalities, and 108 motorcycle fatalities were included. Young men (mean age, 30 years) made up the snowmobile fatalities population, with weekend fatalities predominating (67%). Snowmobile fatalities were associated with use during times of suboptimal lighting (crude odds ratio, 1.9 [95% confidence interval, 1.1–3.3]; P <.01). Blood alcohol concentration exceeded provincial limits in 64% of cases. When snowmobile fatalities were adjusted for occurrence during suboptimal lighting conditions, only alcohol use was associated independently with fatal outcome (adjusted odds ratio, 4.3 [95% confidence interval, 2.5–7.0]; P <.0001).

Conclusion. Drivers in snowmobile fatalities are associated with an approximately fourfold greater use of alcohol than are age- and sex-matched drivers in automobile and motorcycle fatalities.

Do you believe the control group chosen for this study led to bias in the estimate of the size of the association between fatal snowmobile trauma and alcohol use? If yes, why, and would an unbiased estimate be greater or smaller than that obtained by the authors? If not, why not?

Answer 5.6 The control group for this study is comprised of persons with alcohol-related causes of death, in other words, those due to motor vehicle and motorcycle accidents. Therefore, the observed odds ratio is almost certainly lower than the true one.

Question 5.7 Please answer the questions below after reading the following meeting abstract (modified).

Design. Population based case-control study of drivers with known drug and alcohol concentrations who were involved in fatal crashes from October 2001 to September 2003. The cases were the 6766 drivers considered at fault in their crash; the controls were 3006 other drivers.

Results. 681 drivers were positive for cannabis (cases 8.8%, controls 2.8%) (odds ratio 3.32, 95% confidence interval 2.63 to 4.18).

Conclusions. Driving under the influence of cannabis increases the risk of involvement in a crash.

a. Blood specimens were readily available both for cases and controls, and obtaining such specimens on a representative sample of drivers would have posed formidable logistical difficulties. Nonetheless, this choice could have led to a result that was biased to at least some extent.
   i. Under what circumstance(s) would bias arise?
   ii. In what direction would the bias likely be operating, to falsely increase or falsely decrease the odds ratio? Why?

b. In this study, the population attributable risk % (PAR%, the percentage of this population's incidence of a fatal automobile crash attributable to the exposure in question) associated with positive detection of cannabis in blood was 6.1%. The corresponding PAR% for positive detection of alcohol in blood was 28.6%, despite the fact that the proportion of controls in whom each substance was detected was identical. What must be the explanation for the disparity between the size of the PAR% for cannabis and that for alcohol?

Answer 5.7

a. Bias would be present to the extent that the blood levels of tetrahydrocannabinol in drivers killed in auto crashes, who were judged not to be at fault in the crash, did not reflect that of drivers in general. This could occur if either one or both of the following were true:

- The designation of "at fault" sometimes was in error, so that true cases were intermixed into the control group, giving that group a spuriously high proportion of apparent cannabis users.
- Even if not "at fault," drivers who had consumed cannabis were impaired in their ability to avoid a crash.

In either circumstance above, the observed odds ratio associated with evidence of cannabis consumption would be spuriously low.

b. The odds ratio associated with alcohol consumption must have been considerably higher than that for cannabis consumption. (In fact, it was higher: 15.5 vs. 3.3.)

Question 5.8 This question pertains to the following abstract [33]:

Acute influenza infection may be transiently associated with the risk of cardiovascular disease. We examined the association between influenza vaccination and incident myocardial infarction (MI) and stroke in a population-based case-control study. Case subjects were members of Group Health Cooperative (GHC) with incident MI or ischemic stroke during "flu season" (November-March) of 1992–1998. Control subjects were GHC members without history of MI or stroke who were frequency matched to case subjects by age, sex, and calendar year. The medical records of 584 case subjects with MI, 269 case subjects with ischemic stroke, and 1,415 controls were reviewed. Receipt of each year's influenza vaccine was not associated with risk of incident MI (odds ratio [OR] = 0.95, 95% confidence interval [CI]: 0.77, 1.17) or ischemic stroke (OR = 1.20, 95% CI: 0.91, 1.60) during the period of expected influenza activity. This study suggests that . . . influenza vaccination is not associated with a reduction in risk of first MI or ischemic stroke.

By restricting cases of MI and stroke to those that occurred during November-March, the investigators obtained a sample size that was considerably smaller than the one that would have included persons diagnosed with these illnesses in other months as well. What do you believe to have been the primary compensating advantage of the choice they made?

Answer 5.8 It was hypothesized that vaccination might prevent cases of MI and stroke that were precipitated by an influenza infection. Such infections occur primarily in the winter months. The ability of the study to find a true association would have been lessened if MI and stroke cases that were not precipitated by influenza, and thus did not have the potential to be prevented by vaccination, were included. That is, if there truly had been a beneficial impact of vaccination on the risk of MI and/or stroke, the observed odds ratio, using cases in all months, would have been closer to the null than that based on cases diagnosed in November-March.

Question 5.9 The following is excerpted from an article on mesothelioma in relation to employment[34]:

> In a case-control study, the occupational exposures of 259 mesothelioma patients were compared to those of an equal number of controls. Several occupations known to entail substantial exposure to asbestos were more common among cases than controls.

Longest held occupation	Cases	Controls
Insulator	47	13
Shipbuilder	31	21
Plumber	35	28
Furnace or boiler installer or repairman	21	10

> However, there were an identical number of cases and controls (15) who had engaged in brake lining work or repair, indicating that no increase in risk was associated with this type of employment.

Assume the following in this study:

a) Employment status was ascertained without error.
b) Cases and controls were completely comparable with regard to nonoccupational determinants of mesothelioma.
c) Among persons whose longest-held job was not one of the four listed in the above table, those who did brake lining work or repair were no more likely than other persons to also have engaged in one of those four occupations at some time in their lives.
d) Sampling variability is not an issue.

Do you agree with the author's conclusion above regarding the relation of mesothelioma occurrence to brake lining work or repair that was observed in their study? If yes, why? If no, why not?

Answer 5.9 No. To evaluate employment in brake lining work or repair as a possible risk factor for mesothelioma, it is necessary to estimate the mesothelioma incidence in persons with that exposure relative to the risk in a referent category comprised of persons not believed to be at increased risk of this disease. Thus, the analysis should be restricted to persons who had not been employed in furnace and boiler work, insulation, and so forth. If persons who had been insulators, and so forth, had been excluded from the analysis, the referent category would be reduced by 47 + 31 + 35 + 21 = 134 cases and by 13 + 21 + 28 + 10 = 72 controls. The odds ratio associated with employment in brake lining and repair would be as follows:

Brake work	Cases	Controls
+	15	15
−	259 − 15 − 134 = 110	259 − 15 − 72 = 172

$$\text{Odds ratio} = \frac{15}{110} \div \frac{15}{172} = 1.56$$

The authors' interpretation of the results of their study is incorrect.

(It turns out that assumption (c) above is almost certainly not a valid one, i.e., a relatively high proportion of men whose longest held job involved brake lining work or repair indeed had been employed at other times in a high risk occupation. When in a reanalysis attention was restricted to men who had no such history,[37] no greater proportion of mesothelioma cases (1/33) than controls (9/171) had been employed to do brake work.)

Question 5.10 Epidemiologists in California observed that about 65% of infants who died of sudden infant death syndrome (SIDS) typically were put to sleep in the prone position, in contrast to 60% of control infants. Most other studies of SIDS and sleeping position have found a considerably greater case-control difference. Commenting on this result, an editorialist wrote, "One reason that prone sleeping may not have been observed as a strong risk factor for SIDS [in this study] is that it is difficult to measure risk for a characteristic present in 60 percent of the population." Do you agree with this assertion? If yes, why? If not, why not? If not, why not?

Answer 5.10 No, you do not agree.

In terms of the frequency of the exposure, the only circumstance in which case-control studies find "it is difficult to measure risk" is when the exposure either is extremely common (e.g., > 95%) or extremely uncommon (e.g., < 5%). (In those instances, study power is reduced for a given sample size.)

An exposure frequency of 60% is nowhere near these values.

Question 5.11 You have been sent a manuscript to review. It describes the results of a case-control study of gastric ulcer in relation to prior use of nonsteroidal anti-inflammatory drugs (NSAIDS). Cases in this study were all 225 patients diagnosed with a first gastric ulcer between 1982 and 1985 in a given population. All diagnoses were made by endoscopy that had been performed at specialized centers for this purpose. It is believed that gastric endoscopy was not done elsewhere in that part of the world. Community controls were selected randomly from electoral rolls for 1982–1985. After conducting a screening interview with potential control subjects (matched to cases on the basis of sex, age, and area of residence), those with a history of gastric ulcer were excluded. In addition, about 13% of potential controls with dyspepsia were excluded as well: The authors were concerned that: (a) some persons with this symptom might have a gastric ulcer that had not yet been diagnosed; and (b) because NSAID use is a likely cause of dyspepsia, the occurrence of dyspepsia would be considerably more common in NSAID users than in other persons.

Assume that only a very small percentage of those potential controls with dyspepsia actually had a gastric ulcer. Do you agree with the authors' choice to exclude persons with dyspepsia? If yes, why? If no, why not?

Answer 5.11 You disagree. The controls should be a sample of the at-risk population. Cases were included whether or not they had dyspepsia, so persons with dyspepsia were part of the at-risk population. By restricting controls to persons free of dyspepsia, the proportion of persons with a history of use of NSAID would be spuriously low. This would lead to an overestimate of the odds ratio relating a history of NSAID use to the occurrence of gastric ulcer.

Question 5.12 The following is an excerpt from an abstract of a case-control study [35]:

Experimental and epidemiologic evidence has suggested that phenacetin use increases the risk of transitional cell cancers of the urinary tract. The drug is no longer marketed but a commonly used metabolite, acetaminophen, has been linked recently to an increased risk of renal cancer. We assessed the relation of acetaminophen use to the risk of transitional cell cancer of the urinary tract with data from a hospital-based study of cancers and medication use conducted from 1976–96 in the eastern United States. We compared interviews with 498 cases of transitional cell cancer with those of 8,149 non-cancer controls, and controlled confounding factors with logistic regression. For transitional cell cancer, the relative risk (RR) estimate for regular acetaminophen use that had begun at least a year before admission was 1.1 (95% confidence interval (CI = 0.6–1.9). RR estimates for use that lasted at least five years, and for non-regular use, were also close to 1.0. Our results suggest that acetaminophen, as used in present study population, does not influence the risk of transitional cell cancer of the urinary tract.

The authors stated that, in choosing noncancer controls they included only persons hospitalized for conditions that "were judged to be unrelated to acetaminophen use. For example, we did not include patients admitted for gastric or duodenal ulcers, because such persons might have used acetaminophen preferentially to aspirin for pain relief." Do you agree with this strategy? Why? If not, why not?

Answer 5.12 Yes, the strategy is reasonable. By not including patients who were hospitalized because of a condition that is an indication for acetaminophen use, the authors assembled a group of hospitalized patients whose exposure history possibly could reflect that of the source population of the cases. However, it is plausible that a relatively high proportion of hospitalized persons have a history of analgesic use, whether aspirin or acetaminophen. If this is true, the proportion of controls selected for this study who previously had taken acetaminophen would exceed that of the at-risk population, leading to a falsely low odds ratio.

Question 5.13 The following question is based on an excerpt of the abstract of an article "Patent foramen ovale and cryptogenic stroke in older patients"[36]:

> We prospectively examined 503 consecutive patients who had had a stroke, and we compared the 227 patients with cryptogenic stroke and the 276 control patients with stroke of known cause. We examined the prevalence of patent foramen ovale in all patients, using transesophageal echocardiography.
>
> The prevalence of patent foramen ovale [a congenital heart defect] was significantly greater among patients with cryptogenic stroke than among those with stroke of known cause, for both younger patients (43.9% vs. 14.3%; odds ratio, 4.70; 95% confidence interval [CI], 1.89 to 11.68; P<0.001) and older patients (28.3% vs. 11.9%; odds ratio, 2.92; 95% CI, 1.70 to 5.01; P <0.001).

In theory, the control group against which cases of cryptogenic stroke ought to be compared for the prevalence of patent foramen ovale is a sample of persons who are demographically similar to the cases but otherwise unselected. Do you believe that the control group actually chosen in this study correctly produced a positive association between patent foramen ovale and the occurrence of cryptogenic stroke? If yes, why? If no, why not?

Answer 5.13 The control group used—patients with a stroke of "known" cause—will provide a valid result to the extent that the prevalence of patent foramen ovale (PFO) in these persons reflects that of the underlying population from which the cases of cryptogenic stroke arose. *If* the attribution of a known cause had been correct, then a valid result likely would have been obtained, given that there is no reason to believe that the presence of PFO influenced the development of a stroke in these persons. To the extent that some of the cases with a "known" cause were in truth cryptogenic ones, then the observed association between PFO and cryptogenic stroke actually would be spuriously small. (However, the prevalence of PFO in the controls chosen—11.9%–14.3%—was not elevated relative to that expected based on autopsy studies.)

Question 5.14 The following sentence appeared in a review of studies of ovarian cancer incidence in relation to prior use of analgesics: "Three case-control studies observed an inverse association between regular aspirin use and ovarian cancer risk, but in one of these the analysis was based on only one exposed case." Describe a circumstance in which the presence of just one case who took aspirin regularly among a series of cases enrolled in a case-control study of ovarian cancer would argue strongly in support of a beneficial impact of regular aspirin use on risk.

Answer 5.14 The observation would suggest a strong inverse relation if:

a. The total number of women with ovarian cancer and of controls was not too small; and

b. The frequency of aspirin use in controls was high, because this would imply that, in the absence of a true exposure-disease association, the *expected* number of exposed cases would be much greater than 1.

For example:

Regular Aspirin Use	Cases	Controls	Odds Ratio
Yes	1	10	
No	19	10	0.05

Question 5.15 In many instances, ovarian cancer is diagnosed only after the accumulation of a large quantity of fluid in the pelvic cavity that leads to an increase in lower abdominal girth over a period of several months.

A case-control study of ovarian cancer in relation to anthropometric characteristics was conducted in American Medicare-eligible women. Among women diagnosed with ovarian cancer and demographically matched controls with no history of the disease, Medicare records were examined during the three years prior to the date of each case's diagnosis. In the analysis, a comparison was made of the proportion of cases and controls that had "obesity" listed as a diagnostic code in outpatient records at any time in the three-year period. (Typically, a clinical diagnosis of obesity is made on the basis of a very high body weight relative to a person's height.)

The manner in which the presence of obesity was ascertained in the study no doubt led to some degree of misclassification. But apart from this, the design of the study likely led to a spurious estimate of the potential association between obesity and the risk of developing ovarian cancer. Why, and in what direction would the association be biased? Using information available on the study subjects, how might the analysis be reconfigured to provide a more valid estimate?

Answer 5.15 In an ideal epidemiologic study, the presence of obesity would be ascertained prior to the development of ovarian cancer. But in the present case-control study, because of fluid accumulation, the body mass index (as derived from the measurement of weight and height alone) of a given woman with ovarian cancer at the time of diagnosis was likely to have been greater than it was prior to the onset of the malignancy. Therefore, the criterion for obesity in the analysis—being present at **any** time during the three years prior to diagnosis—likely led to an overestimate of the influence of obesity on the occurrence of this disease.

If, in fact, the excess weight accumulated only during a period of several months prior to the diagnosis, the bias could be minimized by considering in the analysis only diagnostic codes for obesity in cases and controls that were assigned before those several months, for example, during just the first two of the three years prior to the date of the case's diagnosis.

Question 5.16 You are planning a case-control study of pneumonia in relation to prior use of medications that reduce gastric acidity (e.g., proton pump inhibitors). The study would take place among members of a large prepaid health insurance plan. You anticipate being able to include as cases all health plan members who were diagnosed with pneumonia during a given period of time, whether or not they required hospitalization for this condition. Use of acid suppressing medications in cases and controls would be ascertained through computerized records of the health plan's pharmacy; the latter is the sole source of medications for most of its members.

You are considering two possible approaches to control definition:

a. A random sample of health plan members who are demographically similar to the cases of pneumonia.
b. (i) For hospitalized cases, health plan members who were hospitalized at the same time for another condition and who also were demographically comparable to the cases. (ii) For outpatient cases, a random sample of demographically comparable health plan members.

Which approach do you prefer? Why?

Answer 5.16 Approach (a) is the one most likely to give a valid result. Because the cases are all those diagnosed with pneumonia in a defined population at risk, as a basis for comparison it is desirable to sample from that same population. Hospitalized patients may differ from persons in the underlying population at risk in terms of use of acid suppressant medications, and conditioning on hospitalization plausibly would give rise to a biased result.

Question 5.17 You have conducted a case-control study of tubal pregnancy, in which a history of prior induced abortion was obtained from cases in a defined population and from a demographically comparable control group of women who gave birth to a child seven to eight months after the cases' diagnoses. Among women with tubal pregnancy, 20% reported having had one or more induced abortions, in contrast to 15% of controls (odds ratio = 1.42).

Before you publish this result, a colleague who has seen data from this same population (see table) cautions that the cases and controls in your study may not have been sufficiently comparable—women who develop a tubal pregnancy typically have it diagnosed and treated quite early in gestation, so that the possibility of an elective abortion in that pregnancy does not arise. She argues that the same is **not** true for women whose pregnancy is intrauterine, and some of them will choose to have the pregnancy aborted and thus not be identified for participation as controls. As shown by the data below, women who have an elective abortion in their current pregnancy are relatively more likely to have had at least one prior abortion in the past. (In the population from which the cases and controls were derived, for every 1000 deliveries there are 308.5 abortions.)

Prior Induced Abortion in Women Undergoing Induced Abortion	
Total	100%
No prior abortions	67.5%
One or more prior abortion	32.5%

You believe your colleague to be correct. In what direction is your original odds ratio biased?

You can calculate an odds ratio that takes this bias into account. What is it?

Answer 5.17 The original odds ratio was falsely high, for controls were women whose frequency of prior induced abortion was falsely low.

The more appropriate control group would include 308.5 women for every 1000 women who had undergone childbirth. The frequency of prior induced abortion in such a group would be:

$$[1000\ (15\%) + 308.5\ (32.5\%)]/1308.5 = 19.1\%$$

The odds ratio would then be:

$$(20/80)/(19.1/80.9) = 1.06,$$

in contrast to the odds ratio of 1.42 that was obtained when the controls were restricted to women who had undergone childbirth.

Question 5.18 In a study of 73 men with testicular tumors who had been born with undescended testicles, 14 had previously undergone an orchiopexy (an operation to bring the testicles into the scrotum). All orchiopexies had taken place between 11 and 36 years of age.

Because it is well established from other work that men born with undescended testicles are at a large increased risk of developing a testicular tumor, the authors of the study concluded that in a boy with undescended testicles an orchiopexy should be performed prior to 11 years of age. What additional data are needed in men without testicular tumors to justify this recommendation?

Answer 5.18 Without information on receipt of—and age at—orchiopexy among men without testicular tumors who were born with undescended testicles, it cannot be known whether an orchiopexy during boyhood has the ability to lessen the cancer risk. A very different conclusion would be drawn if (say) 50% of men in that population without testicular cancer born with undescended testicles had undergone orchiopexy prior to age 11—a result suggesting considerable efficacy of the procedure against cancer occurrence—than if the figure were zero percent (i.e., the same percentage as in the cases of testicular cancer).

Question 5.19 The text below is taken from an Abstract of an article in the American Journal of Epidemiology (2011; 174:451–8):

> The authors evaluated indoor air pollution from coal combustion (IAPCC) as a potential risk factor for neural tube defects (NTDs) in a rural population in Shanxi Province, China. The studied rural population has both high IAPCC exposure and a high prevalence of NTDs. A population-based case-control study was used to identify 610 NTD cases and 837 liveborn controls between November 2002 and December 2007. Information was collected within one week following delivery or pregnancy termination due to prenatal NTD diagnosis. The authors derived an exposure index by integrating a series of IAPCC-related characteristics concerning dwelling and lifestyle.

In this study, the cases were a mixture of infants born with an NTD and aborted fetuses with an NTD. All controls were live born infants. Do you believe the more valid comparison would restrict cases and controls to those who were live born, or rather the comparison chosen by the authors in which no such restriction was made?

Answer 5.19 Excluding NTD cases who were aborted would to some extent produce a case-control study of risk factors for not receiving prenatal NTD screening. The inclusion of all NTD cases, aborted or live born, is likely to provide a more valid evaluation of risk factors for NTDs.

Question 5.20 A study was conducted in a part of the world where polio has not yet been eradicated, in order to estimate the efficacy of oral polio vaccine (OPV). From children with acute flaccid paralysis, two stool samples were obtained within 14 days of the onset of symptoms, and then tested for the presence of poliovirus. Parents of children who tested positive on at least one sample (cases) and negative on both samples (controls) were queried regarding immunization histories of the children. The results were as follows:

Receipt of OPV	Cases	Controls
Yes	160	90
No	40	10

Although the examination of stool for the presence of poliovirus is believed to be 100% specific—no false positives—it probably is not 100% sensitive. Assume that among the 100 controls in the study, 10% truly were cases, irrespective of vaccination history. Estimate the vaccine effectiveness in the presence and the absence of this misclassification.

Answer 5.20

The odds ratio based on the original 100 controls is $\dfrac{160}{40} \div \dfrac{90}{10} = 0.444$, and the vaccine effectiveness would be estimated as $\dfrac{(1/.444)-1}{1/.444} \times 100\% = 55.6\%$.

Now suppose that among the 100 controls, 10 children (10%) were actually misclassified cases. Among these 10, the prevalence of OPV exposure should be the same as that among the cases already identified, that is, 160/200 = 80%. Hence we would expect 10 * 80% = 8 of the misclassified cases to have had OPV vaccination, and the other 2 would not. Had these 10 misclassified cases been shifted from the control group to the case group, the results would have looked like this:

OPV	Cases	Controls
+	160 + 8 = 168	90 – 8 = 82
–	40 + 2 = 42	10 – 2 = 8

The odds ratio with this source of misclassification removed would be (168/42)/(82/8) = 0.39, and the corresponding estimate of vaccine effectiveness would be $\dfrac{(1/.390)-1}{1/.390} \times 100\% = 61.0\%$.

The imperfect ability to distinguish cases from controls would lead to an underestimate of the ability of OPV immunization to prevent polio.

Question 5.21 A study was conducted to gauge the possible role of cannabis use in motor vehicle collisions.[38] Among 368 drivers of automobiles involved in a collision, a blood sample was obtained within six hours and tested for the presence of a metabolite of cannabis. The proportion of the drivers who tested positive was compared to the proportion who claimed to have used cannabis within six hours prior to the time they had previously driven. About one in five of the study subjects had evidence of the cannabis metabolite in their blood, a far higher proportion than would have been expected based on the proportion who claimed to have used cannabis in the six hours before the earlier driving episode (matched odds ratio = 12.0).

Based on the different sources from which cannabis use was ascertained, you are concerned that the design of this study could have led to a spuriously large association of recent cannabis use with collision risk. Why?

Answer 5.21 In this analysis, the means of exposure assessment were not comparable for the two periods of time: blood metabolite levels for the "case" period, recall for the "control" period. Incomplete ascertainment of cannabis use during the control period by means of an interview would have led to a falsely large estimate of the association.

(Indeed, the authors provide some evidence that the interview did not accurately elicit use: In reporting on their use of cannabis within six hours of the collision, nearly half of the persons with metabolites identified in blood claimed no recent use.)

Question 5.22 A group of investigators reviewed the charts of 3800 American men who sought an evaluation for infertility, and identified 10 in whom a testicular cancer had been found during the evaluation (six by means of physical examination, four by means of testicular ultrasound). To determine the expected frequency, they obtained the incidence of testicular cancer among demographically similar men from U.S. population-based cancer registries.

Would you expect this comparison to provide a valid result? If yes, why? If no, why not?

Answer 5.22 The investigator's comparison of testicular cancer prevalence (among the infertile men studied) and incidence (from registry data) produced a result that is uninterpretable. What is needed as a basis for comparison is an estimate of the prevalence of as-yet-undiagnosed testicular cancer in men without infertility.

Question 5.23 A colleague from the Department of Dermatology has brought you the data below. They come from a small case-control study of melanoma of the head and neck. Each melanoma case was matched to 10 controls of the same sex who had other skin problems. All study subjects were then asked about prior use of hair dye. The dermatologist wishes to know whether he must control for the variable "sex" or, having matched on it, he can now ignore it. What is your answer, and how would you support it quantitatively?

Hair dye	Men	
	Cases	Controls
Yes	2	11
No	9	99
Total	11	110

Hair dye	Women	
	Cases	Controls
Yes	12	96
No	4	64
Total	16	160

Answer 5.23 Matching in a case-control study precludes using study data to evaluate whether the matching factor is truly a confounder in the source population from which cases and controls were drawn. This is because the matched controls are not necessarily a representative sample of all non-cases in the source population: the frequency of exposure among them may be skewed by differential selection according to a matching factor that may be correlated with exposure. Even if the matching factor is unrelated to disease among unexposed persons in the source population (so that it cannot be a confounder), it may nonetheless behave as a confounder in a matched case-control study if it is associated with exposure.

In this example, even though we cannot determine whether sex is truly a confounder in the source population, sex does behave as a confounder in the study data:

- A higher proportion of women than men had used hair dye; and
- Within strata of hair dye use, there were different proportions of men and women between cases and controls.

The sex-specific odds ratios each are 2.0, and so the unconfounded odds ratio would be 2.0. But the crude odds ratio actually is

$$(14 / 13) / (97 / 163) = 1.64$$

In order to avoid bias (the above pattern of associations could be due to confounding, or just to differential selection of controls by sex, or to both), the variable "sex" needs to be controlled for.

CHAPTER 6

Multiple Causal Pathways and Effect Modification

AN IMPORTANT THREAT to an epidemiologic study's sensitivity in identifying a genuine exposure–disease association is error in the measurement of the exposure and/or the illness outcome. Confounding can be another threat. A third, not as widely appreciated as measurement error and confounding, is a study's failure to take into account the presence of causal pathways leading to disease other than the one under consideration. The means by which these other pathways can be accommodated vary from study to study. Sometimes, illness outcomes can be subdivided based on the presence or absence of a manifestation of the condition in question, for example, estrogen receptor-positive breast cancer from estrogen receptor-negative breast cancer in studies of hormonal exposures. Alternatively, persons in whom a known potent etiologic agent is present can be omitted from consideration, so as to allow the influence of an exposure acting to cause disease through a different means to be seen (e.g., in studies of mental retardation, when children with microcephaly are excluded when studying the potential influence of postnatal exposure to low levels of metals in the environment). However, interpreting the results of analyses based on subgroups of the study population is not always straightforward—as we'll see in some of the following examples.

Question 6.1 You come across an abstract of an article in a medical journal, which in part reads as follows:

> In our study of women diagnosed with endometrial cancer, possible risk factors were identified through personal interviews. Among women with endometrial cancer who had and had not taken unopposed estrogen therapy prior to the time the tumor was diagnosed, there were no differences with regard to parity [i.e., the number of children they had borne]. The results of this study do not support the hypothesis that parity is differentially associated with endometrial cancer that is and is not related to exogenous estrogens.

Based on the above summary, what do you believe to be the main limitation of this study in evaluating whether parity has a different relationship to the etiology of endometrial cancer that is and is not related to unopposed estrogen use?

Answer 6.1 The differential relationship between a particular characteristic of a woman's reproductive history and endometrial cancer, according to a history of estrogen use, can be discerned only by measuring the size of the association between that characteristic and endometrial cancer in estrogen users and then again in nonusers. Since no comparison group is mentioned, the presence of an association cannot be assessed in either group of women.

Question 6.2 Persons with a factor V Leiden mutation are resistant to the anticoagulant effect of activated protein C. The following table describes the incidence of first venous thrombosis (VT) in women ages 15 to 49 years, according to presence of the factor V Leiden mutation and the use of oral contraceptives (OC):

	Cases of VT	Person-years	Incidence of VT per 10,000 person-years
Factor V Leiden negative			
No OC use	36	437, 870	0.8
Current OC use	84	275, 858	3.0
Factor V Leiden positive			
No OC use	10	17, 515	5.7
Current OC use	25	8757	28.5

Assume that the incidence of first and recurrent VT bear a similar relation to oral contraceptive use and the factor V Leiden mutation. In a 15- to 49-year-old woman who develops VT, do the data presented above argue that her factor V Leiden status should be considered in counseling about her future method of contraception?

Answer 6.2

Factor V Leiden	Incidence of VT per 10,000 person-years	Rate ratio	Rate difference per 10,000 person-years
Negative			
No OC	0.8		
Current OC	3.0	3.7	2.2
Positive			
No OC	5.4		
Current	28.2	5.0	22.8

Yes. Although OC use is associated with an increased incidence of VT regardless of factor V Leiden mutation status, the recommendation is supported by the considerably larger absolute increase in the rate of VT associated with OC use in factor V Leiden-positive than in factor V Leiden-negative women: 22.8 per 10,000 person-years versus 2.2 per 10,000 person-years.

Question 6.3 A study observed that, for a given history of cigarette smoking, the relative risk for lung cancer among women was 1.2- to 1.7-fold greater than it was in men. The disparity between the sexes was well beyond that expected by chance, and led the authors to conclude that women were more susceptible than men to respiratory carcinogenesis from cigarette smoke.

A subsequent letter to the editor of the journal in which the article was published suggested that in order to use the data from the study to infer differential susceptibility between the sexes, it would be necessary to know the incidence of lung cancer in men who had not smoked and in women who had not smoked. Why would this additional information be useful?

Answer 6.3 If the rate in female nonsmokers were lower than in male nonsmokers, the same added risk associated with cigarette smoking in the two sexes would produce a larger relative risk in women.

For example:

	Incidence in nonsmokers*	Incidence in smokers*	Attributable risk*	Relative risk
Men	10	30	20	3
Women	5	25	20	5

*Rate per 100,000 person-years.

Therefore, depending on how *differential susceptibility* is defined—greater relative risk versus greater attributable risk—women and men may or may not differ in terms of the impact of smoking on their incidence of lung cancer.

Question 6.4 This question pertains to the following excerpt of an abstract[39]:

> *Background.* Elderly people who have a fracture are at high risk of another. Vitamin D and calcium supplements are often recommended for fracture prevention. We aimed to assess whether vitamin D3 and calcium, either alone or in combination, were effective in prevention of secondary fractures.

> *Methods.* In a factorial-design trial, 5,292 people aged 70 years or older (4481 [85%] of whom were women) who were mobile before developing a low-trauma fracture were randomly assigned 800 IU daily oral vitamin D3, 1000 mg calcium, oral vitamin D3 (800 IU per day) combined with calcium (1000 mg per day), or placebo. Participants who were recruited in 21 UK hospitals were followed up for between 24 months and 62 months. Analysis was by intention-to-treat and the primary outcome was a low-energy fracture.

In their trial, the investigators identified 698 participants in whom a "low-energy" fracture occurred. Not included in the analysis were an additional 34 fractures that resulted from substantial trauma, for example, a fracture sustained in an automobile crash.

The disadvantage of not including the 34 fractures involving more than a low level of trauma is a reduced sample size (by about 5%). What do you believe to be the main advantage of this choice?

Answer 6.4 The investigators believed that the relative influence of one or more of the intervention measures on the risk of fracture could differ depending on the level of trauma to which a participant was exposed. If very little trauma were present, the relative benefit might be great; in the presence of substantial trauma, there might be but little benefit from the intervention. Therefore, to maximize the sensitivity of the study to observe any relative change in fracture occurrence associated with one or more treatments, the analysis excluded persons with fracture in whom another factor, substantial trauma, likely played a causal role.

Question 6.5 You observe that among persons 20 years of age or older who developed a particular infectious disease, 32% had been vaccinated against that disease, in contrast to 16% of persons under 20 years with the disease. Is this necessarily evidence of greater vaccine efficacy in younger persons?

Answer 6.5 No, such a conclusion would not be justified. In order to assess vaccine efficacy in either age group, it would be necessary to estimate the percentage of the population at risk who had been vaccinated.

	<20		≥20	
Vaccinated	Cases	Population	Cases	Population
Yes	32%	?	16%	?
No	68%	?	84%	?

Question 6.6 In a study of the possible adverse effect of the drug rosuvastatin on the incidence of venous thromboembolism (VTE),[40] the investigators separately analyzed "provoked" and "unprovoked" cases. "Provoked" cases were defined as those in which a strong risk factor had been present, such as recent surgery, immobility or metastatic cancer. What do you believe to have been the rationale for making this separation?

Answer 6.6 If rosuvastatin acted together with other VTE risk factors in a causal pathway, the size of the association might have been expected to be particularly great for "provoked" cases. Alternatively, if the means by which rosuvastatin predisposed to VTE were independent of other risk factors, the relative risk associated with its use would be expected to be greatest for unprovoked VTE. An analysis that examines each type of VTE separately enables the evaluation of either possibility.

Question 6.7 The data presented in the table below appeared in a publication of the results of a case-control study on the risk of endometrial cancer in relation to physical activity and obesity.[41] Based on the data in the table, the authors stated that "the increase in risk associated with obesity [BMI ≥30] was much lower in active women (OR = 1.57) than in women with low physical activity (OR = 3.10)." What is a more accurate way of quantifying the difference in the relative risk of endometrial cancer associated with BMI ≥30 within the two categories of physical activity? Why might the approach used by the authors be misleading?

Lifetime physical activity and endometrial cancer risk, by BMI

	Average lifetime physical activity					
	Low			High		
BMI	Cases	Controls	OR (95% CI)†	Cases	Controls	OR (95% CI)†
<25	105	100	1.0	59	74	0.95 (0.57–1.58)
25–29	81	72	1.0	52	84	0.58 (0.34–0.99)
≥30	113	49	1.0	62	64	0.50 (0.28–0.91)
<25	105	100	1.0	59	74	0.90 (0.56–1.43)
25–29	81	72	1.39 (0.88–2.20)	52	84	0.85 (0.52–1.38)
≥30	113	49	3.10 (1.91–5.01)	62	64	1.57 (0.94–2.62)

*Below and above the median.
†Odds ratio (OR) and 95% CI were adjusted for age, race/ethnicity, education, family history of endometrial cancer, age at menarche, full-term pregnancies, duration of oral contraceptive use, duration of hormone therapy use, menopausal status, and height.

Answer 6.7 We wish to know whether the size of the OR associated with a high BMI on risk differs according to physical activity. Among less active women, the OR associated with obesity is 3.1. Among more active women, it is 1.57/0.90 = 1.74. (The OR of 1.57 incorporates *both* the elevated risk associated with obesity and the reduced risk associated with activity.)

Question 6.8 In a cohort study, postmenopausal women who were taking combined estrogen-progestogen hormone therapy at baseline had a 5-year cumulative incidence of breast cancer of 5.6/1,000 if their mother had a history of breast cancer, and 2.2/1,000 if not. Among hormone nonusers, the corresponding cumulative incidences were 5.1/1,000 and 1.7/1,000, respectively.

a. Among women with a maternal history of breast cancer, what was the relative risk of breast cancer associated with use of hormone therapy at baseline? The risk difference?

b. What were these same measures of excess risk in women without a maternal history of breast cancer?

c. The two means of assessing the potentially modifying influence of maternal breast cancer on the association between hormone use and risk of breast cancer do not produce the same qualitative result. Why is this?

You are trying to decide whether to differentially counsel postmenopausal women with and without a maternal history of breast cancer with regard to the impact of hormone therapy (perhaps in terms of the frequency of breast screening exams). Which contrast do you believe to be the most relevant for this purpose, the one between the two relative risks or that between the two risk differences? Explain.

Answer 6.8 a.

Maternal history	Relative risk	Risk difference (per 1,000)
+	5.6 per 1000/5.1 per 1000 = 1.1	5.6 – 5.1 = 0.5
–	2.2 per 1000/1.7 per 1000 = 1.3	2.2 – 1.7 = 0.5

b. In this instance, the same absolute increase in risk associated with hormone therapy (0.5/1,000) is acting upon a smaller background risk in women without a positive maternal history, producing a greater relative change in their risk (1.3) than the relative change (1.1) in women with a positive maternal history.

c. The size of the absolute change in risk associated with hormone therapy is what bears on personal decision making. Because the additional risk associated with hormone therapy is 0.5/1,000 irrespective of maternal history, counseling should not be differential between the two groups of women with regard to actions that might be taken.

Question 6.9 A study was conducted in sub-Saharan Africa among heterosexual couples in whom just one member was infected with HIV.[42] During the course of a 24-month follow-up, about 10% of participants who were infected at baseline initiated antiretroviral therapy. The study observed that among persons who were HIV-negative at baseline, the acquisition of an HIV infection that was phylogenetically linked to that of their HIV-infected partner was relatively less common among those whose partners had received antiretroviral therapy (0.37 vs. 2.24 per 100 person-years).

Had the study endpoint been *any* new HIV infection, irrespective of its linkage to the HIV strain of the initially infected partner (so as to include HIV infections that arose from sexual contact with other persons), what would have been the expected impact (if any) on the following measures of association:

a) Rate difference
b) Rate ratio

Explain.

Answer 6.9 If receipt of antiretroviral therapy by one's HIV-infected partner were unrelated to the likelihood of acquiring an HIV infection from a different partner, then the size of the absolute increase in the incidence of any new HIV infection above that of the "linked" infections would be the same whether or not antiretroviral therapy had been administered. In this circumstance, the rate difference would be unchanged, but the rate ratio associated with the partner's receipt of antiretroviral therapy would be closer to the null.

For example, assume an incidence of "unlinked" HIV infection in initially HIV-negative persons of 0.20 per 100 person-years:

Type of HIV infection	Antiretroviral treatment		Rate difference (per 100 person-years)	Rate ratio
	Yes	No		
Linked	0.37	2.24	1.87	6.1
Unlinked	0.20	0.20	0	1.0
Total	0.57	2.44	1.87	4.3

The presence of a second causal factor leading to disease (in this instance, sexual contact with another HIV-infected person)—one that does not join with the first factor in an etiologic pathway and is not accounted for in the study design and/or analysis—will lead to an attenuation of the estimated rate ratio of the disease associated with the first causal factor.

Question 6.10 The following letter, somewhat paraphrased, appeared in a medical journal:

> Bailar and Gornik report that the age-adjusted rate of mortality from all cancers in the United States declined by 1 percent from 1991 through 1994. Our estimate for the same interval is 2.2 percent. The discrepancy in the two figures stems from the use of different populations for age adjustment. Bailar and Gornik used the relatively elderly 1990 U.S. population and by doing so, minimized striking reductions in mortality that occurred among young and middle-aged persons. We used the U.S. (relatively younger) 1940 population, which reveals the full downturn in cancer-related mortality.

Suppose that you also are interested in quantifying the change in U.S. cancer mortality during 1991-1994, and have access to age-specific U.S. mortality rates for those years. In your analysis, would there be any virtue in presenting adjusted rates within specific age categories (e.g., "young and middle-aged" versus "older")? If yes, why? If no, why not?

Answer 6.10 Yes, there would be value in presenting age-specific rates. During the 4-year period under study there was, apparently, a "striking reduction" in cancer mortality in the United States in young and middle-aged persons, but not in older persons. Only the presentation of age-specific differences over time can illustrate this difference in trends. A measure such as a difference in adjusted rates across all ages will provide a summary that may not apply to any individual age group. Furthermore, as is clear from the letter to the editor, the size of the mortality trend will be influenced by the arbitrary choice of the age distribution to be used as the standard.

Question 6.11 The following is an abstract of an article "Occupational asbestos exposure and the incidence of non-Hodgkin lymphoma of the gastrointestinal tract: An ecologic study."[43]

> *Purpose.* A previous case-control study observed a strong association between occupational exposure to asbestos and the incidence of non-Hodgkin lymphoma of the gastrointestinal tract (GINHL). To test this hypothesis we sought to determine whether the geographic pattern of the incidence of GINHL in the US has paralleled that of mesothelioma.

> *Methods.* Using data obtained from the nine US regions participating in the National Cancer Institute's Surveillance, Epidemiology, and End Results program, we examined the incidence of malignancies among men ages 50 to 84 years between 1973 and 1984.

> *Results.* The rates of mesothelioma, but not of GINHL, were about two times higher in the areas of Seattle and San Francisco than in the other regions. Overall, there was no correlation between the rates of mesothelioma and of GIHNL (Person correlation coefficient—0.12, $\rho = 0.77$).

> *Conclusions.* This ecologic study finds no support for the hypothesis that occupational asbestos exposure is related to the subsequent incidence of GINHL.

In their analysis, the authors paid particular attention to rates in men (in whom the likelihood of prior occupational exposure was far greater than in women) and to rates in 50- to 84-year-olds (to allow for a potentially long induction period). And, even though the Surveillance, Epidemiology, and End Results program had data available through the 1990s, the authors confined their analysis to cancer incidence through just 1984. What do you believe to have been their reason for this latter choice? (Hint: The presence of HIV infection strongly predisposes to the development of GINHL.)

Answer 6.11 GINHL has a number of causal pathways that may lead to its occurrence. One of these involves HIV infection. If occupational asbestos exposure adds to a person's risk of GINHL to the same extent whether HIV infection is present or not, then the relative increase in risk associated with asbestos exposure will be greatest in HIV-uninfected persons. Therefore, the most sensitive assessment of the potential role of asbestos is to exclude cases related to HIV. One way of accomplishing this is to restrict the time period being considered to that before HIV infection was widespread, in other words, prior to 1985.

(Because the prevalence of HIV infection varies geographically across the United States, failure to control for HIV infection in this way also could lead to confounding. For example, GINHL rates in San Francisco during the last decade of the twentieth century might be high relative to other parts of the United States because of the relatively high prevalence of HIV infection there, and not because of a higher degree of occupational asbestos exposure.)

Question 6.12 A study sought to determine if pregnancy intendedness is associated with intimate-partner physical violence, and to identify factors that modify this association. Three to 6 months after delivery, the investigators mailed a questionnaire to a population-based sample of 12,612 mothers of infants born in four states.

Some of the results of this study are shown in the following table:

Percentage of women experiencing physical violence during pregnancy, by pregnancy intendedness and education

Education (y)	Unwanted		Intended	
	%	(95% CI)	%	(95% CI)
All	12.1	(8.8–15.6)	3.2	(2.4–4.0)
<12	18.6	(9.6–27.6)	7.0	(4.1–9.9)
12	10.6	(5.9–15.3)	3.7	(2.5–4.9)
>12	9.2	(2.7–15.7)	1.3	(0.7–1.9)

The authors stated that the risk for experiencing violence in women who had an unwanted pregnancy, relative to the risk in women with an intended pregnancy, was particularly high among women with more social advantage. For example, the relative prevalence among women with fewer than 12 years of education was 2.6, whereas the corresponding relative prevalence in women with >12 years of education 7.1.

In discussing the findings, the authors put forth some possible explanations "for the interaction between pregnancy intendedness, social status, and physical violence." Could it be argued that, apart from the issue of chance (i.e., sampling variability), there is *no* interaction to account for? If yes, why? If no, why not?

Answer 6.12 The investigators used a relative measure of association to assess the possibility of an "interaction" between education and pregnancy intendedness as a predictor of physical violence. However, the data suggest that, in absolute terms, the increased risk of experiencing violence associated with an unwanted versus an intended pregnancy is about the same for all levels of education. If anything, the observed difference in prevalence was greater in women with <12 years of education (18.6% – 7.0% = 11.6%) than in women with >12 years of education (9.2% – 1.3% = 7.9%).

Question 6.13 The data presented in the following table are from a hypothetical study of perinatal death among twins in relation to order of delivery.*,†

| Gestational age (weeks) | No. of twin pregnancies | No. of perinatal deaths in: | | b/a |
		first-born twin (a)	second-born twin (b)	
24–27	703	359	381	1.06
28–31	1,371	98	141	1.44
32–35	2,897	74	164	2.22
≥36	2,935	33	124	3.76

Would it be reasonable to infer from these results that the increase in risk of perinatal death in the second-born twin is a particular concern in a term or a near-term pregnancy, and less so in a pregnancy that ends well prior to term? Explain.

---

* Infants born to women undergoing a planned caesarean section are excluded.
† Restricted to pairs in which at least one twin survived.

Answer 6.13 At gestational ages 24–27 weeks, the risk of perinatal death in first-born twins is 359/703 = 51/100, and that in second-born twins is 381/703 = 54/100. The difference in risk of death between second- and first-delivered twins at other gestational ages also is about 3 per 100. Therefore, although the relative difference in risk of death differs across gestational age categories, the added risk among second-delivered twins is of similar concern irrespective of gestational age.

| Gestational age (weeks) | Risk of perinatal death (per 100) | | Relative risk | Risk difference (per 100) |
	First-born twin	Second-born twin		
24–27	51.1	54.2	1.06	3.1
28–31	7.1	10.3	1.45	3.2
32–35	2.6	5.7	2.19	3.1
≥36	1.1	4.2	3.82	3.1

Question 6.14 The following is adapted from a report of a case-control study of primary liver cancer in relation to serum levels of retinol, in which serum samples had been obtained prior to the diagnosis of cancer.[44]

> Men with low prediagnostic serum retinol levels had a relatively high risk of liver cancer. A statistically significant interaction was observed between retinol levels and hepatitis B surface antigen (HBsAg) seropositivity on cancer risk: HBsAg-positive men in the lowest third of the distribution of serum retinol had greater than a 70-fold higher risk than HBsAg-negative men in the highest third of the distribution of serum retinol (p for interaction = .018).

From the information provided, can you determine the nature of the interaction between retinol levels and HBsAg status with regard to the incidence of liver cancer? If yes, what is it? If not, what additional information from the study would you need?

Answer 6.14 No, the nature of the interaction cannot be determined. In each of the following examples, assume (for simplicity) that the odds ratio associated with the presence of both low retinol levels and HBsAg+ relative to high retinol levels and HBsAg– is not 70, but instead is 100 (200/100 ÷ 20/1000), based on the hypothetical data shown below.

The risk of liver cancer associated with low retinol levels might be particularly great in men who are HBsAg positive:

	HBsAg+			HBsAg–	
	Case	Control		Case	Control
Low retinol	200	100	Low retinol	700	1000
High retinol	10	100	High retinol	20	1000
Odds ratio	20				3.5

Or, it might not:

	HBsAg+			HBsAg–	
	Case	Control		Case	Control
Low retinol	200	100	Low retinol	700	1000
High retinol	10	100	High retinol	20	1000
Odds ratio	20				35

Only in the first example is the odds ratio associated with low retinol levels greater in HBsAg+ men than HBsAg– men. Therefore, what's needed to understand the nature of the interaction is the size of the odds ratio (or the risk difference, if examining a deviation from additivity) associated with retinol levels within categories of HBsAg seropositivity.

Question 6.15 The following data come from a case-control study of upper gastrointestinal bleeding (UGIB) in relation to prior use of nonsteroidal anti-inflammatory drugs (NSAIDS).

History of ulcer	NSAID use	Cases	Controls
No	No	607	15,242
No	Yes	171	597
Yes	No	405	1,430
Yes	Yes	106	164

Do the data from this study suggest that, when deciding to initiate treatment with an NSAID, the risk of UGIB should weigh less heavily as a potential adverse effect in persons with a history of an ulcer than in other persons? Explain your answer.

Answer 6.15 The decision to use an NSAID (or any other drug) should be based in part on a comparison of the size of the added benefits and added risks that such use would entail. From the data obtained in this case-control study, it is possible to estimate the relative risk of UGIB (by means of the odds ratio) but not the added ("attributable") risk. Nonetheless, the relative size of the added risk associated with NSAID use in persons with, and in persons without, a history of ulcer can be calculated, as shown below:

Ulcer	NSAIDS	Cases	Controls	Odds ratioa	Odds ratiob	Relative added risk
No	No	607	15,242	1	1	7.19 – 1 = 6.19
No	Yes	171	597	7.19	7.19	
Yes	No	405	1,430	1	7.11	16.23 – 7.11 = 9.12
Yes	Yes	106	164	2.28	16.23	

[a] Separate referent category of nonusers of NSAIDs for persons with and without a history of ulcer.
[b] Common referent category = Persons with neither a history of ulcer nor of NSAID use.

The relative added risks associated with use of an NSAID obtained above have no units, but nonetheless can be meaningfully compared between persons with and without ulcers. Since the added risk of UGIB incurred as a result of NSAID use is similar in the two groups (if anything, it is greater in those *with* ulcers [i.e., 9.12 vs. 6.19]), it should receive equal weight by potential NSAID users irrespective of ulcer history. The fact that the first odds ratio is so much smaller in patients with ulcers than in patients without ulcers is attributable to the higher underlying rate of UGIB in ulcer patients.

Question 6.16 The following data were obtained in a very large cohort study conducted in Korea during 1993–2002 that examined potential risk factors (including the prevalence of hepatitis B surface antigen positivity (HbsAg+)) for mortality from hepatocellular carcinoma (HCC).

	# of HCC cases	Rate per 100,000 person-years
Men		
HbsAg+	1522	405.2
HbsAg-	734	21.8
Women		
HbsAg+	37	58.2
HbsAg-	9	1.2

a. For men and women, separately, estimate the relative mortality from HCC associated with being HBsAg+, and also the mortality difference.
b. One of the above measures of excess mortality is greater in men; the other is greater in women. How can this be?

Answer 6.16

a. Relative mortality
    Men: 405.2 /21.8 = 18.6
    Women: 58.4/1.2 = 48.7

    Mortality difference (per 100,000 person-years)

    Men: 405.2–21.8 = 383.4
    Women: 58.4–1.2 = 57.2

b. The annual mortality from HCC, in the absence of active infection with hepatitis B, differs greatly by sex: 21.8 per 10^5 in men versus 1.2 per 10^5 in women. Thus, even a moderate absolute increase in mortality of 57.2 per 10^5 experienced by Korean women corresponds to a very large increase in relative terms (RR = 48.7). In men, the much larger absolute mortality difference (383.4 per 10^5) is not nearly so large, relatively speaking, because it is superimposed on the higher male "baseline" rate of 21.8 per 10^5.

Question 6.17 The following is an excerpt from a school of public health alumni magazine:

> Knowing your blood type may help you manage your risk for heart disease. People with type AB, B, or A may be more vulnerable—with type AB linked to the highest risk (20% increase). [The author of the study] said, 'If you know you're at higher risk [based on ABO blood type], you can reduce the risk by eating right, exercising, and not smoking.'

Knowledge of ABO blood type probably should have NO influence on how a person manages his/her risk of heart disease. Why?

Answer 6.17 Do "eating right, exercising, and not smoking" have little or no impact on the risk of heart disease in persons with *type O* blood? Only if this were true—which is unlikely, and in any case not addressed in the data provided—would it be appropriate for knowledge of blood type "to help you manage your risk."

Question 6.18 A meta-analysis of published studies of tobacco smoking in relation to the incidence of nasopharyngeal cancer (NPC) obtained a relative risk of 1.60 associated with ever having smoked. This value differed, however, according to the underlying incidence in the population under study. In the United States and Europe, where the incidence of NPC in nonsmokers is about one per 100,000 per year, the relative risk was 1.76. In Asia, where the incidence of NPC in nonsmokers is about 10 per 100,000 per year, the relative risk was just 1.29. Assume that the associations observed in the meta-analysis are indicative of a causal influence of tobacco smoking on the occurrence of NPC.

The authors concluded that "tobacco smoking may have a greater impact on NPC risk among populations in low-risk areas than among populations in high-risk areas." Estimate the NPC incidence among smokers of tobacco attributable to their smoking in low- and high-risk populations. Do you agree with the authors' conclusions?

Answer 6.18

The incidence of NPC attributable to cigarette smoking can be estimated as follows:

Population	Incidence in Nonsmokers*	Relative Risk	Incidence in Smokers*	Attributable Rate*
Low-risk	1	1.76	1.76	0.76
High-risk	10	1.29	12.90	2.90

*per 100,000 per year

In absolute terms, the impact of tobacco smoking is, if anything, greater in high-risk than in low-risk populations.

Question 6.19 In many persons, bisphosphonate medications can prevent bone loss associated with aging, and in randomized trials use of these drugs is associated with a reduced incidence of fractures of the femur. Based on some case reports, however, there is concern that bisphosphonate use might predispose users to a certain rare type of femoral fracture ("atypical" fracture), which has distinctive radiologic features.

In a case-control study designed to examine the question of bisphosphonate use as a risk factor for atypical femoral fracture, both the cases and members of the ideal control group would have had an indication for use of these drugs, such as a history of a skeletal fracture or of a bone scan indicating the presence of bone thinning. Because it can be difficult in practice to enumerate potential controls meeting this criterion, an investigator chose instead persons who had sustained a femoral fracture that was *not* atypical. Although such a choice did provide a control group that was comparable to the cases in terms of having a predisposition to fracture, it nonetheless would be expected to lead to a biased result. Why, and in which direction?

Answer 6.19 Use of bisphosphonates reduces the incidence of femoral fractures as a whole, and so must reduce the incidence of "typical" femoral fractures (given that these comprise the large majority of femoral fractures). Therefore, even if bisphosphonate treatment truly had no influence on the incidence of *atypical* femoral fractures, a higher proportion of persons with atypical fractures would have a history of use of these drugs relative to persons with other femoral fractures, leading to a spuriously high risk estimate.

Question 6.20 A collaborative group of investigators conducted a randomized trial of the efficacy of an human papillomavirus (HPV) vaccine against the development of anal intraepithelial neoplasia (AIN, a precursor of anal cancer) in gay men.[45] Participants were assigned to receive three doses of a *quadrivalent* vaccine (directed against HPV types 6, 11, 16, and 18) or a placebo, and were examined for the presence of AIN approximately three years following receipt of vaccine or placebo.

Among men in the treatment arm of the trial, there were 74 cases of AIN in 569.0 man-years of follow-up. The corresponding numbers in the placebo group were 103 cases in 588.4 man-years.

a. What was the efficacy of the vaccine against the presence of AIN?

b. The tumors of about 60% of the cases of AIN among participants in the trial contained DNA from HPV 6, 11, 16, or 18, whereas the other cases had DNA of other HPV types present. Had the study outcome been restricted to AIN in which HPV 6, 11, 16, or 18 had been present, would you expect the estimate of efficacy to have been the same, higher, or lower than that calculated in (a)? Explain. (Assume that the vaccine used had no impact on the occurrence of AIN from HPV types other than 6, 11, 16, and 18.)

Answer 6.20

a. $\text{Vaccine efficacy} = \dfrac{103/588.4 - 74/569}{103/588.4} \times 100\%$

$= \dfrac{.175 - .130}{.175} \times 100\% = 25.7\%$

b. The absolute incidence of AIN resulting from an HPV infection that was not type 6, 11, 16, or 18 would be expected to be identical between vaccine and placebo groups. Therefore, the relative difference in the incidence of AIN that *did* contain HPV 6, 11, 16, or 18 should be greater in this second analysis, leading to an increase in the estimate of vaccine efficacy, and this is exactly what was observed.

Question 6.21 In a study of 985 women treated for endometrial cancer at a large American medical center during 1999–2009, the mean age at diagnosis decreased steadily across categories of body mass index, from 67.1 years in the leanest women to 56.3 years in the most obese.[46] Cognizant of prior research documenting the strong association between obesity and the risk of endometrial cancer, the authors concluded that "as obesity becomes more severe, the underlying carcinogenic mechanisms cause endometrial cancer earlier in women's lives." What is your principal reservation concerning the authors' conclusion?

Answer 6.21 The observed pattern could well be attributable to a difference in the distribution of body mass index according to age in the underlying population, and have nothing to do with endometrial cancer at all. Such a difference could be due to one or both of the following: (1) the large increase in the average body mass index of American women over successive birth cohorts in the 20th century; and (2) the increased mortality from other causes associated with a very high body mass index. In order to assess the possible difference in the etiologic role of obesity in the development of endometrial cancer at various ages, it would be necessary to compare the size of the relative or attributable risk associated with obesity across age groups.

Question 6.22 Investigators in New Zealand conducted a study to determine whether home modifications intended to decrease the incidence of falls (e.g., stair rails, bathroom grab rails, slip-resistant surfacing of decks and porches) could lead to a decrease in injuries from falls.[47] Residents of 842 households agreed to be subject to random assignment for a home evaluation, with modifications as needed either made immediately (intervention arm) or delayed three years (control arm). Records of a personal injury insurer that covered the residences were examined for the three-year period following the time the home modifications began (and the corresponding time period for control households) for claims for unintentional home injuries.

Using text descriptions of the injury, and without knowledge of the intervention status of the household, the investigators judged the cause of the injury to be fall-related or not, and then judged whether the fall occurred in circumstances that could have been prevented by one or more of the home modifications available. (For example, if a slip or fall occurred while gardening or as a result of tripping over a toy, it was deemed not preventable by the modifications.)

A total of 182 injuries from falls were reported in the 950 residents of the households in which modifications were made, in contrast to 192 in the 898 residents of control households. Taking into account the person-time at risk, this corresponded to a rate ratio of 0.86, and a rate difference of 11 injuries from falls per 1000 person-years.

When attention in the analysis was restricted to the injuries from falls that were classified as being potentially preventable as a result of home modifications, would you expect the (a) rate ratio; and (b) rate difference to differ from these figures? Explain.

Answer 6.22 Assuming that the home modifications had no impact on the incidence of injuries from gardening, tripping over toys, etc., the rate ratio in the second analysis (that excluded such injuries) would be expected to be lower, that is, to be indicative of a greater reduction in risk. Indeed, this is what was observed in the study: a rate ratio of 0.66 was observed. Exclusion of causal pathways to fall injury apart from those that the modifications were designed to eliminate led to a more sensitive assessment of the intervention's impact.

In contrast, the rate difference would be expected to be virtually unchanged (as it turned out to be: 10 per 1000 person-years in the second analysis versus 11 per 1000 person-years in the first analysis), given that the initial analysis had already captured all of the absolute change in incidence that occurred.

Question 6.23 The relative risk of hepatocellular carcinoma associated with chronic infection with hepatitis B virus is about 200 in Taiwan, whereas in Greece it is about 10. Yet the attributable rate (excess cases per 100,000 person-years) in persons residing in these two countries is nearly identical. How is this possible?

Answer 6.23 The prevalence of other causal pathways leading to hepatocellular carcinoma must be higher in Greece than in Taiwan. In other words, the risk of this disease in persons who are not chronically infected with hepatitis B virus must be higher in residents of Greece than in residents of Taiwan.

The relative and attributable risks presented might have come from the following sets of incidence rates in the two countries:

| | Annual Incidence per 100,000 | | | |
	Infected	Uninfected	Relative risk	Attributable risk per 100,000
Greece	440	44	10	396
Taiwan	400	2	200	398

Question 6.24 A concern occasionally is expressed that though most medical research focuses on disease, people are interested primarily in health. This has led some to recommend the conduct of studies evaluating the role of one or more interventions in producing and maintaining a person's health.

You suspect that it might be difficult to operationalize the definition of "health" in a particular study. Still, for the moment assume that in such a study no misclassification would be present—healthy and unhealthy persons could be identified without error. Also, assume that the study could be configured so as to eliminate confounding when examining the possible influence of a given intervention. Nonetheless, you believe that the ability of the study to identify a genuine impact of the intervention on health, broadly defined, could be quite limited. Why is this?

Answer 6.24 There can be many bases for a person being unhealthy. If one of these is uncommon, even something that is completely effective at preventing it may have but a small influence on the likelihood of being healthy. For example, assume that the presence of a chronic toothache is responsible for 1% of individuals who are not in good health, but that access to high-quality dental care can successfully deal with pain from this source in every instance. The risk of being "unhealthy" among persons with high-quality dental care would be 1% lower than among persons without such access. It is the rare epidemiologic study, however, that is large enough (and is adequately free of confounding) to identify convincingly a 1% reduction in risk.

Note that in a study not of health, but rather of chronic dental pain, in the above scenario the relative risk associated with access to high-quality dental care would be zero and not 0.99. The focus on the more narrowly defined outcome of chronic dental pain allows for attention to be focused on the one causal pathway leading to being "unhealthy" to which the lack of high-quality dental care can contribute, and, therefore, provides a greater ability to identify a salutary impact of high-quality dental care.

CHAPTER 7

Screening

AT A POPULATION LEVEL, the degree to which a screening test can lead to improved health outcomes is related to:

a. The proportion of the population with the condition (or predictor of that condition) that the test seeks to detect;
b. The sensitivity of the test in identifying the condition or predictor;
c. A low frequency of false positive tests, or a low frequency of adverse health outcomes associated with the consequences of a false positive test; and
d. The efficacy of treatment of persons who screen as positive.

Often, elements a-d above are addressed in separate studies. Occasionally, though, especially when we don't have available to us the experience of untreated persons who have tested positive, a single study seeks to examine the aggregate impact of two or more elements (e.g., a comparison of cancer mortality in screened and unscreened persons). The exercises in this chapter consider studies of the individual elements as well as those that deal with several of these at once.

Question 7.1 In 132 patients with cirrhosis of the liver, serum levels of alpha-L-fucosidase were measured and the patients were followed for 8 years for the occurrence of liver cancer. In 12 of them, levels of this enzyme were "high." Liver cancer was diagnosed in 19 patients, and in 3 of the 19, serum alpha-L-fucosidase levels were "high."

a. From the data provided, calculate the
   1. Sensitivity
   2. Specificity
   3. Predictive value of a positive test
   4. Predictive value of a negative test
   of a "high" level of serum alpha-L-fucosidase in patents with cirrhosis for predicting liver cancer during the ensuing eight years.

b. There was a "significant increase" 6 to 9 months before evidence of liver cancer in 7 of the 16 patients who had low serum levels of alpha-L-fucosidase at enrollment. What other information is needed before concluding that a change of this sort is useful in predicting the presence of liver cancer?

c. The authors of this paper concluded, "We recommend the measurement of this enzyme activity in surveillance programs for cirrhotic patients." Even if the serum alpha-L-fucosidase level in a person with cirrhosis perfectly discriminated between those who did and did not develop liver cancer, is it possible that this recommendation could be misguided? How?

Answer 7.1

"High activity"	Cancer	No cancer	Total
Yes	3	9	12
No	16	104	120
	19	113	132

a. 1. Sensitivity = 3/19 = 0.16
   2. Specificity = 104/113 = 0.92
   3. PV+ = 3/12 = 0.25
   4. PV– = 104/120 = 0.87
b. Other information needed: In what proportion of patients who did not develop liver cancer was there a "significant increase" in levels?
c. The recommendation could be misguided if, on average, early recognition of a liver tumor, by means of this test, did not result in an improved outcome.

Question 7.2 The following appeared in the "News" section of the *Journal of the National Cancer Institute*, May 17, 2000:

Some Promising Biomarkers for Cancer
- **LPA (lysophosphatidic acid).** "LPA is probably the most accurate marker we have for detection of early stage ovarian cancer," said Northwestern University's David Fishman, M.D., who is heading a multi-center study of the marker. A 1998 report from the Cleveland Clinic found 9 of 10 women with stage 1 disease, 24 of 24 with advanced disease, and 14 of 14 with recurrent ovarian cancer had elevated blood LPA levels. In contrast, just 5 of 48 controls had elevated LPA. A growth factor, LPA is not generally present in normal ovary cells.

Based on the above information, you believe it *un*likely that blood LPA levels will be of practical use in the early detection of ovarian cancer. What is your reasoning?

Answer 7.2 If the prevalence of ovarian cancer among screened women is low, the number of false positive tests— many of which would lead to a surgical procedure to document the absence of ovarian cancer—would greatly exceed the number of true positives. If the prevalence of cancer is 1/2,000, for example, these would be the expected results in 20,000 screened women:

LPA	Ovarian cancer		Total
	Yes	No	
Positive	10	5/48 (19,990) = 2,082	2,092
Negative	0	43/48 (19,990) = 17,908	19,990
	10	19,990	20,000

The PV+ would be 10/2,092 = 0.005, very likely too low to warrant use of LPA for early detection. For conditions whose prevalence is relatively low, this question illustrates the strong influence of a test's specificity on the predictive value of a positive test result.

Question 7.3 A test was developed (based on levels of a certain peptide in blood) to identify persons with congestive heart failure. After studies revealed that a negative test predicts the absence of heart failure virtually 100% of the time, the manufacturer of the test concluded that a positive test is "an unambiguous warning sign" for the presence of congestive heart failure. You disagree. Why?

Answer 7.3

	Congestive heart failure		
Test Results	Yes	No	Total
+	A	b	a + b
−	c (0%)	d (100%)	c + d

In order for a positive test to represent "an unambiguous warning sign," its positive predictive value (a/(a + b)) would have to be high. However, the presence of a negative predictive value (d/(c + d)) of 100% does not speak to this issue.

Question 7.4 The questions below pertain to the following abstract (abridged):

Survival of Women Ages 40-49 Years with Breast Carcinoma according to Method of Detection

Methods. Women ages 40-49 years diagnosed with invasive breast carcinoma between 1986 and 1992 were identified. Measures of tumor size, lymph node status, and overall survival were compared with breast carcinoma patients whose tumors were detected by breast self-exam (BSE), clinical breast exam (CBE), patient incidental finding (PI), or mammography.

Results. Mean tumor size among women in the mammography group was smaller than that among women in the BSE, CBE, and PI groups (*P* <0.002).Tumors detected by mammography were significantly more likely to be localized than those detected by other methods (*P* <0.0001). Patients whose tumors were detected by mammography had significantly better survival than patients in the other detection method (*P* <0.0001).

Conclusions. Women ages 40-49 years whose invasive breast carcinoma is detected by mammography have significantly smaller tumors, more localized disease, and may have a lower risk of mortality than women whose tumors are detected by other methods.[48]

a. When interpreting their findings, the authors of the study discussed the possibility of lead-time bias accounting for the relatively better survival of women whose breast cancer was detected by means of screening mammography. Why might lead-time bias have been present?
b. To address this concern, the authors adjusted for tumor size and extent of disease when comparing survival across the groups of women with breast cancer defined by method of detection. What is the primary limitation of an analysis of this sort?

Answer 7.4

a. Mammography is a relatively more sensitive means of breast cancer detection: It can identify cancers earlier in their natural history than can self-exam or clinical exam. Therefore, even if there were no effective treatment for early breast cancer, the mean interval from diagnosis to death would be greatest in women whose tumors were identified via mammography, due to their added "lead-time" prior to the age they otherwise would have been diagnosed. In the absence of effective treatment, receipt of screening mammography would not have extended life, but rather it would have extended that portion of the same life span during which a woman was known to have breast cancer.

b. Screening has the potential to exert a favorable influence on the likelihood of cancer mortality only by identifying tumors that are relatively early in their natural history, in other words, small in size and limited in their spread. Adjusting for these characteristics would not allow whatever true benefit that screening has on survival to be evident.

Question 7.5 This question pertains to the following news article that appeared in the April 20, 2005, issue of the *Journal of the National Cancer Institute*:

> **Group Recommends Earlier Colorectal Cancer Screening for African Americans**
>
> The American College of Gastroenterology has recommended that physicians begin screening African Americans for colorectal cancer at age 45 rather than at age 50, the general recommendation made by several groups.
>
> In the publication of the recommendation, which appears in the March issue of the *American Journal of Gastroenterology*, the authors point out that African Americans have the highest incidence of colorectal cancer of any racial or ethnic group. In addition, they note that the mean age of presentation among African Americans is lower than whites.

The American College of Gastroenterology based its recommendation (regarding a racial difference in the age at which screening for colorectal cancer begins) on the high incidence and low mean age at presentation of colorectal cancer in African Americans. The latter is *not* a valid reason. Why?

Answer 7.5 It is possible that the basis for the relatively younger age distribution of African-American cases is the relatively younger age distribution of African Americans in general. The incidence rate of colorectal cancer among 45- to 49-year-olds—the relevant piece of data that would bear on the recommendation—could be identical between the races and the mean age at diagnosis would still be lower in African Americans than in whites.

Question 7.6 The following is excerpted from the abstract of an article on computer-aided detection of early breast cancer.[49]

> We determined the association between the use of computer-aided detection at mammography facilities and the performance of screening mammography from 1998 through 2002 at 43 facilities in three states. We had complete data for 222,135 women (a total of 429,345 mammograms), including 2351 women who received a diagnosis of breast cancer within 1 year after screening. We calculated the specificity, sensitivity, and positive predictive value of screening mammography with and without computer-aided detection.
>
> Diagnostic specificity decreased from 90.2% before implementation to 87.2% after implementation ($P < 0.001$). The increase in sensitivity from 80.4% before implementation of computer-aided detection to 84.0% after implementation was not significant ($P = 0.32$).
>
> The use of computer-aided detection is associated with reduced accuracy of interpretation of screening mammograms. The increased rate of biopsy with the use of computer-aided detection is not clearly associated with improved detection of invasive breast cancer.

The size of the decrease in specificity associated with computer-aided detection—90.2% – 87.2% = 3.0%—was slightly smaller than the size of the increase in sensitivity—84.0% – 80.4% = 3.6%. However, the p value for the difference in specificity (<0.001) was far smaller than that for the difference in sensitivity (0.32). What is the reason for the disparity between the size of two p values?

Answer 7.6 The calculation of the specificity is based on the women without breast cancer, whereas the calculation of the sensitivity is based on the women with breast cancer. The p value is heavily influenced by the number of subjects, and in this study the women without cancer outnumbered the women with cancer by nearly 100 to 1. Thus, the p value must be smaller for the difference in specificity than that for the difference in sensitivity.

Question 7.7 A randomized trial of fecal occult blood screening for colorectal cancer was conducted in Minnesota.[50]

a. During a follow-up period of 18 years, the incidence of colorectal cancer that was first diagnosed when metastatic (stage D) in 15,570 persons assigned to annual screening was only 53% that of 15,394 persons assigned to not be screened; for 15,587 persons assigned to be screened every 2 years, the corresponding figure was 68%. Are any other data needed to show that screening was successful?

b. The table below summarizes the mortality experience of the three study groups. In assessing the efficacy of fecal occult blood screening, should attention be focused primarily on total mortality or mortality from colorectal cancer?

	Study group		
	Annual screening	Biennial screening	Control
No. enrolled	15,570	15,587	15,394
Person-years of observation	240,325	240,163	237,420
Deaths from all causes			
No. of deaths	5,236	5,213	5,186
Cumulative mortality*	342	340	343
95% confidence interval (CI)	334–350	333–348	336–531
Deaths from colorectal cancer (CRC)			
No. of deaths	121	148	177
Cumulative mortality*	9.46	11.19	14.09
95% CI	7.75–11.17	9.39–12.99	12.01–16.17

* Per 1000.

Answer 7.7

a. The answer depends on the criterion for success. On average, persons in the groups assigned to receive screening did have their tumors detected at a relatively earlier stage than persons assigned not to be screened. However, unless treatment at this earlier stage is more efficacious than that given later, no lives will have been saved. Therefore, if one wishes to learn whether screening led to a reduction in mortality, it is necessary to compare mortality rates in the screened and unscreened participants.

b. If assessment of cause of death is believed to be largely unaffected by screening history and the impact of screening is believed to be confined to averting deaths from colorectal cancer, then the focus of the analysis should be on mortality from colorectal cancer. If there are potentially fatal complications of the screening process (e.g., perforated colon during colonoscopy that would follow a positive stool exam) or treatment (e.g., death during cancer surgery), deaths from these causes should be included as well.

A comparison of all-cause mortality would be an insensitive means of measuring the potential benefit associated with screening: Even if annual screening prevented *every* death from colorectal cancer and had no bearing on any other cause of death, the all-cause mortality in the screened group would be decreased by only 3% $\left(\dfrac{5,186-177}{5,186} = 0.97 \right)$

Question 7.8 The following is excerpted from a manuscript describing the results of a cohort study of screening for stomach cancer (by means of photofluorography, a highly sensitive test) in Japan in relation to mortality from stomach cancer:

> The present study focused on 100,562 subjects who were ages 40–79 years at the time of a baseline survey, which asked for their screening experience during the past twelve months. Of these, 219 subjects with a history of stomach cancer prior to the time of the baseline survey were excluded, as were 8,386 subjects who did not provide information on their participation in stomach-cancer screening.
>
> Death rates from stomach cancer during a period following the baseline survey, adjusted for differences in age and other demographic characteristics, were compared between participants with and without a history of screening for this disease.

Do you believe this study is likely to provide a valid estimate of the ability of screening photofluorography to lead to a reduction in mortality from stomach cancer? If yes, why? If not, why not, and in which direction do you believe the bias will occur?

Answer 7.8 The design of this study does not permit an unbiased estimate of the potential impact of photofluorographic screening on mortality from stomach cancer. The problem stems from what has been referred to as "healthy screenee bias."[28] The "exposed" cohort in the present study has received a screening exam in the prior year that was negative: Had it been positive for cancer, such persons would have been removed from the cohort. The "unexposed" cohort has not had such persons identified or excluded. Thus, even if screening led to completely ineffective treatment, or to no treatment at all, the observed relative mortality from stomach cancer would be lower in the screened group.

Question 7.9 You find the following in an article in a medical journal:

> Pap smear screening may be less effective among black women than among white women. Laboratory-based evidence of Pap smear screening (i.e., a Pap smear performed in the absence of symptoms of cervical cancer) at least once during the past 5 years was found for 48% of the black population with invasive cervical cancer versus only 32% of the white population with invasive cervical cancer ($p < 0.05$).

Assuming that ascertainment of invasive cervical cancer was equally complete for the black and white populations and that management of the Pap smear abnormalities was similar for the two groups, what reason might there be for the observed result other than a differential effectiveness of Pap smear screening between the two races?

Answer 7.9 It is possible that in the underlying population from which the women with cervical cancer were drawn, a higher percentage of black women than white women had undergone Pap screening at least once in the past 5 years. What is needed in order to gauge the efficacy of this screening modality in the prevention of invasive cervical cancer is the proportion of women in the population at risk who had been screened. Suppose the following results would have been observed in a case-control study of invasive cervical cancer:

	Black women		White women	
	Invasive cancer	Controls	Invasive cancer	Controls
% screened	48	60	32	44
% not screened	52	40	68	56
Odds ratio	0.6		0.6	

In this situation, the relative impact of screening in reducing the incidence of invasive cervical cancer would have been identical in black and in white women.

Question 7.10 A randomized trial was performed to determine whether screening women with ovarian cancer in clinical remission for serum levels of a tumor marker every 3 months, followed by treatment of recurrences identified through this means, could reduce mortality. Women were recruited into the trial at the onset of the remission induced by their initial treatment. Those who later were found to have elevated levels of the marker were randomized to one of two approaches to management:

(a) Immediate chemotherapy; or
(b) No additional treatment until the recurrence became apparent for other reasons (typically, the development of symptoms), on average 5 months later. (Values for serum levels of the tumor marker in patients in group (b) were not provided to these women's physicians.)

In comparing mortality between women in groups (a) and (b), should rates be calculated from the time of randomization or from the time of recognition of the recurrence? Explain the reason for your answer.

Answer 7.10 The mortality rates in both groups should be based on follow-up beginning at the time of randomization, in other words, when the elevation in serum levels of the tumor marker was first apparent. Follow-up beginning at the time of recognition of the recurrence would give rise to lead-time bias: Only in group (a) would person-time be accrued during (on average) the first 5 months after tumor marker elevation was noted, and in this period of time mortality from ovarian cancer would be expected to be considerably smaller than in the period following symptom development.

(A randomized trial of the efficacy of screening for the tumor marker CA 125, designed in the manner described in this question, did indeed tabulate mortality rates in both groups from the time of randomization.[54])

Question 7.11 You are designing a case-control study to estimate the efficacy of PSA screening for prostate cancer. From
the records of a large prepaid health-care plan, you are going
to ascertain screening histories of men who died as a result of
prostate cancer during 2007-2009. As a basis for comparison,
you are considering two possible control groups (who would be
individually matched to the fatal cases):

1. Members of the health-care plan who are demographically comparable to the fatal cases and also were diagnosed with prostate cancer at about the same time,
   but who were still alive at the time of the matched
   case's death
2. Demographically comparable members of the health
   plan who had not been diagnosed with prostate cancer
   as of the date of diagnosis of their matched fatal case

Which of the two groups above would provide the more
valid result? Explain.

Answer 7.11 Option 2 conforms to the goal of control definition, in other words, a sample of the population from which the cases were derived. The problem with option 1 is that, even if no effective treatment were available for screen-detected prostate cancer (in which case the correct odds ratio should be one), there would be a higher proportion of screened men in controls than cases (assuming that PSA screening has some sensitivity for detecting prostate cancer).[55]

Question 7.12 A case-control study was conducted to assess the impact of cervical screening in reducing the incidence of invasive cervical cancer.[51] Because such screening can identify cervical precancerous lesions, it was hypothesized that a smaller proportion of cases than controls would have been screened at some point during the prior 4 years.

The women with cervical cancer had been diagnosed during 2000–2003; they were identified using records of a cancer registry serving the area in which the study was done. The receipt of screening during 1996–2003 was ascertained by means of a registry that enumerated screening exams in that area. Age-matched controls were chosen from women identified in the screening registry during 1996–2004. The investigators explained that "each case would still have the possibility of being matched to control(s) with no screening history prior to the case's diagnosis," since some controls would have received their first screen during 2004 and so would have been unscreened during 1996–2003.

What do you perceive to be the greatest threat to the validity of this study?

Answer 7.12 The purpose of a control group in a case-control study is to estimate the proportion of "exposed" persons in the population (who were at risk of the disease in question) from which the cases arose. In this instance, the investigators needed screening histories on a sample of women with a cervix who resided in the area from which the cases had been derived. It would be fortuitous if the sampling from the controls who were chosen by the investigators succeeded in accomplishing this. Almost certainly, the level of screening in the controls actually selected (from a screening registry) overstated that in the population at risk, leading to an observed odds ratio (approximately 0.1) that was falsely low.

Question 7.13 Hackam et al. ascertained prior use of anti-hypertensive and other medications among patients over 65 years of age hospitalized with a ruptured abdominal aortic aneurysm ("cases," n = 3,379) and those hospitalized with an unruptured aneurysm ("controls," n = 11,947).[52] In the course of reviewing electronic files of medical services that preceded the aneurysm diagnosis, the investigators incidentally noted receipt of abdominal imaging (ultrasound, CT, or MRI) in nearly all of the patients with an unruptured abdominal aortic aneurysm, but in only a small fraction of those with a ruptured aneurysm.

Screening by means of abdominal imaging has the potential to lead to identification of an aortic aneurysm, and in turn to surgical intervention that could avert a rupture. However, despite the large observed case-control difference in the prior receipt of screening by means of abdominal imaging, it would *not* be appropriate to use the data of Hackam et al. to support the hypothesis that screening could lead to a reduced risk of a ruptured abdominal aortic aneurysm. Why? What would be a better basis for comparison to the patients with a ruptured abdominal aortic aneurysm?

Answer 7.13 In order for a case-control study of screening efficacy to provide a valid result, the level of screening in the controls must reflect that of the population at risk from which the cases were derived. All of the controls in this study were known to have an abdominal aortic aneurysm, many, no doubt, as a result of screening, and so the level of screening in them would be expected to be atypically high. Thus, even if there truly were no beneficial impact of early recognition and treatment of abdominal aortic aneurysms on the occurrence of rupture, a (far) smaller proportion of persons with a ruptured aneurysm than a known unruptured one would have a history of screening.

If one were to design a case-control study to estimate the ability of aneurysm screening to reduce the occurrence of ruptured abdominal aortic aneurysm (this was not the goal of Hackam et al.), controls would need to be selected from an entirely different sampling frame. If (as in this study) the cases of ruptured aneurysm were all those over age 65 diagnosed in a specific geographic population, the controls ideally would be demographically similar members of that same population.

(Fortunately, there are data available from randomized trials from which we can gauge the efficacy of ultrasound screening for abdominal aortic aneurysm.[56])

Question 7.14 In order to gauge the efficacy of screening by means of a digital rectal exam (DRE) or measurement of levels of prostate-specific antigen (PSA) in serum against mortality from prostate cancer, a case-control study was conducted.[46] A comparison was made between receipt of either of these screening modalities in 74 men who died as a result of prostate cancer ("cases") and in a sample of year-of-birth matched men who resided in the same county as did the cases. Because of the concern that tests performed close to the time of the diagnosis of prostate cancer might have been prompted by symptoms, the primary analysis focused on screening tests performed during the 1 to 5 years prior to diagnosis of prostate cancer, and during the corresponding period of time in control men. Screening tests had been performed on 81.3% of controls during this interval, in contrast to just 60.8% of the fatal cases (odds ratio = 0.35, 95% confidence interval = 0.17–0.71).

Because of the means by which "exposure" was defined in the primary analysis, it is likely that a smaller proportion of cases than controls would have been screened, even had early identification of prostate cancer failed to lead to treatment that would favorably influence the risk of death from prostate cancer. Why is this?

Answer 7.14 For a screening modality that is sensitive (such as a serum PSA measurement for the presence of prostate cancer), excluding the 12 months prior to diagnosis from consideration will effectively exclude most positive tests. And, because positive tests are proportionally far more numerous in men with prostate cancer than in men in general, exclusion of the 12 months prior to diagnosis means that proportionally more cases than controls who had been screened will be classified as not having been screened. Therefore, even if screening failed to lead to any mortality reduction, this analytic approach would give rise to an odds ratio less than 1, suggesting efficacy against cancer mortality when in truth none had been present.

A valid result in case-control study of screening requires accurate assessment of receipt of screening in cases and controls during the whole of the period prior to diagnosis or symptoms (whichever comes first) that correspond to the period of potential detectability.[57]

Question 7.15 A physician was bemoaning the declining use of prostate-specific antigen (PSA) screening for prostate cancer in the United States during the past several years. He had believed there would be negative "public health repercussions" as a result of the decline, and saw evidence of this in the following national data: fewer prostate biopsies being performed, fewer prostate cancers found and, when found, the tumors were on average more aggressive than when PSA screening had been more prevalent.

You do not believe these trends necessarily represent a negative public health repercussion. Why?

Answer 7.15 A *negative* public health repercussion would be an increase in the RATE of aggressive prostate cancer in the United States. But from the evidence provided, it is possible that this rate actually has been steady, and the increasing PROPORTION of aggressive disease among the prostate tumors found is due only to a decline in the rate of nonaggressive tumors that have been diagnosed. Given the morbidity associated with treatment of nonaggressive prostate tumors and the limited efficacy of that treatment, the observed trend actually may represent a positive repercussion of a decline in screening.

Question 7.16 A group of investigators sought to document the incidence of breast cancer within a year following a negative screening mammographic examination. Among approximately 200,000 women who took part in a screening program in a U.S. metropolitan area during the 1990s, they identified those who were diagnosed with breast cancer (and whose cancer was reported to a population-based cancer registry serving that area) during the 12 months following each woman's last negative exam. (There was an average of 2.0 screening mammograms per woman during the period of the study.) The observed incidence of breast cancer was 29.5 per 10,000 during the year following the most recent negative exam.

Assume that there has been no misclassification of the screening status of the mammograms performed in the study population, and that all incident cancers were successfully ascertained. The figure of 29.5 per 10,000 is an overestimate of the incidence of breast cancer in screen-negative women during the following year. Why is this? What do you believe would be a better estimate of that incidence?

Answer 7.16 The failure to consider the incidence of "interval" breast cancer after ALL negative screens, and not just the most recent one, has led to an inflated estimate of risk. The incidence of breast cancer during the year following any earlier negative screen must have been zero, given that screening is provided only to women without a history of breast cancer. Given that women had, on average, exactly two exams during the study period, the incidence of breast cancer during the one-year period following a negative screen is exactly half of 29.5 per 10,000, that is, 14.75 per 10,000 women.

Question 7.17 Adult-onset diabetics have about twice the mortality rate as nondiabetics. A trial was mounted to determine whether screening for the presence of diabetes would lead to treatment that would reduce this difference. Among 19,226 residents of Great Britain not known to have diabetes, 15,089 were assigned at random to be invited for screening for blood glucose and HbA1c (a marker of longer-term glucose levels). Potential cases were evaluated by means of an oral glucose tolerance test, and those confirmed as being diabetic were entered into an aggressive treatment program. The remaining 4137 patients did not undergo screening.

During an average follow-up of 9.6 years, 3% of patients in the group assigned to be screened were diagnosed with diabetes. The primary outcome measure employed by the investigators, the all-cause mortality rate, was no lower in the intervention group (10.5 per 1000 person-years) than among patients in the control arm of the trial (9.9 per 1000 person-years, 95% CI of the relative mortality = 0.90–1.25).

a. One factor that limited the ability of the trial to document a health benefit from screening was the substantial fraction—27%—of persons in the intervention arm who did not respond to the invitation to be screened. What was (likely) an even more important factor? Explain.

b. The authors of the article reporting the results of this study acknowledged the failure of the intervention to lead to a decrease in all-cause mortality in the screened population, and suggested that the benefits of screening may be restricted to the diabetics themselves. From the data gathered in the study, it would be straightforward to compare all-cause mortality in persons after a diagnosis of diabetes in the intervention and control arms of the trial. However, even if there truly were no mortality reduction resulting from screening, such an analysis almost certainly would observe a lower all-cause mortality rate among intervention-arm diabetics than among the control-arm diabetics. Why?

Answer 7.17

a. The potential contribution of screening to the prevention of all-cause mortality in the entire screened population is quite small. If diabetics constitute 3% of the population, a relative mortality of two means that deaths among them would constitute some 6% of deaths. Even if screening prevented all excess deaths among diabetics, which is not likely, only 6–3 = 3 of every 100 deaths would be prevented. The resulting mortality ratio of (100–3)/100 = 0.97 would be difficult-to-impossible for any trial to identify reliably.

b. The presence of lead-time bias would distort the truth. In participants in the intervention arm, diabetes would be identified earlier in its natural history than in their counterparts in the control arm. Even if screening did not influence the natural history, the additional person-time accrued in screen-detected diabetics would produce a lower mortality rate than in diabetics whose condition was detected (later on, on average) by other means.

Question 7.18 In a randomized trial of the effectiveness of prostate specific antigen (PSA) screening, mortality from prostate cancer was reduced by 20% (p < .01). However, no significant difference in all-cause mortality was observed. A commentator suggested that "the benefit of early diagnosis could be offset by the complications from the diagnostic test and subsequent treatment," and that "men may be trading one cause of death for another."

What reservation do you have with the interpretation that PSA screening leads to the death of some men from causes other than prostate cancer?

Answer 7.18 It may be that there is a true decrease in all-cause mortality associated with receipt of PSA screening, but that the trial did not have the statistical power to document this. Because mortality from prostate cancer is but a small fraction of that mortality, even a 100% reduction in deaths from prostate cancer might reduce total mortality by too small a proportion to be detectable in all but the very largest study.

Question 7.19 In an effort to reduce mortality from cutaneous melanoma, dermatologists and public health workers in one state in Germany mounted a campaign intended to lead to earlier diagnoses. Through mass media and informational leaflets sent by insurers, residents of the state were encouraged to see their physician or a dermatologist for a skin exam. Immediately prior to this time, the majority of physicians practicing in the state were provided with a day's instruction on the conduct of skin exams.

Approximately 360,000 persons > 20 years of age, some 19% of the state's adult population, sought a skin exam from a physician during 2003–2004. By 2010, the mortality from cutaneous melanoma in the state had fallen by 48% from precampaign levels. In contrast, there was no corresponding decline in any of four neighboring states in which no similar campaign had been undertaken.

Assume that the between-state difference noted above was neither the result of chance nor confounding. Nonetheless, you have a reservation regarding the authors' interpretation of these results as indicating efficacy of screening for cutaneous melanoma. What is that reservation?

Answer 7.19 Many of the exams performed likely were not strictly "screening" exams, but rather were visits by persons with a suspicious skin lesion who saw a physician about this due to prompting by the campaign. Evidence to support this hypothesis comes from the disparity between the proportion attending an exam—19%—and the 48% reduction in mortality. Almost certainly the difference is due to the selective nature of the patients seen, that is, those with skin lesions that they had noticed. Whether screening per se—that is, an exam of a person with no knowledge of any skin lesions—leads to a reduction in melanoma mortality cannot be gauged from this study.

Question 7.20 Mesothelioma is a rare malignancy that most often arises in pleural tissue (the lining of the lung). Its first clinical manifestation typically is a pleural effusion (the presence of fluid in the pleural cavity), though pleural effusions can occur for other reasons as well. In many persons with pleural mesothelioma, there is a history of heavy occupational asbestos exposure. Nonetheless, among persons who had been heavily exposed to asbestos the prevalence of as-yet-undiagnosed mesothelioma is estimated to be only about 1 in 200. In persons who had been heavily exposed to asbestos who now have a pleural effusion, in some 10% the effusion is the result of a pleural mesothelioma.

A comparison of persons with and without mesothelioma for a plasma level of a substance called fibulin-3 of > 52.8 mg/mL observed a sensitivity of 96.7% and a specificity of 95%. These values were the same whether the comparison group was asbestos-exposed persons in general or asbestos-exposed persons with a pleural effusion for other reasons.

Based on these results, it is likely that the measurement of plasma fibulin-3 levels in persons with occupational exposure to asbestos has the potential to be of clinical utility in the diagnosis of mesothelioma among persons with a pleural effusion, but less so in predicting which asymptomatic asbestos-exposed person has pleural mesothelioma. Why?

Answer 7.20 The predictive value (PV+) of this test will be far greater when used in asbestos-exposed persons with a pleural effusion—in whom the prevalence of mesothelioma would be relatively high (10%)—than in asbestos-exposed persons in general, in whom but one in 200 would have the disease.

All Asbestos-exposed Persons	Fibulin-3	Yes	No		PV+
	> 52.8	967	6567	7534	12.8%
	≤ 52.8	33	192,433	192,466	
		1000	199,000	200,000	
Pleural Effusion Present		Yes	No		
	> 52.8	967	297	1264	76.5%
	≤ 52.8	33	8703	8736	
		1000	9000	10,000	

Question 7.21 A group of investigators sought to determine the extent to which the presence of the tumor antigen CA-125 predicted the presence of ovarian cancer before it became symptomatic. In a cohort of healthy women on whom blood samples had been obtained at cohort entry, they identified participants who were diagnosed with ovarian cancer during the following three years. In serum from the initial blood draw, 57% of these women had levels of CA-125 that exceeded 35 U/mL. Only 2.4% of women who did not develop ovarian cancer during the three-year period had a "baseline" serum CA-125 level that was greater than 35 U/mL.

Despite the strong association observed, the authors cautioned against using serum CA-125 levels as a screening test for ovarian cancer, because the test was "not sufficiently sensitive." You believe there is a better reason for being pessimistic regarding the potential utility of serum CA-125 levels as a screening test for occult ovarian cancer. What is it?

Answer 7.21 The predictive value of a positive CA-125 test is likely to be quite low: Because only a tiny fraction of asymptomatic women will have ovarian cancer, in absolute terms, 2.4% times the large number of non-cases is likely to be far greater than 57% times the small number of cases.

A sensitivity of less than 100%, even far less, is not necessarily an important consideration in gauging the potential utility of a screening test. If the test under consideration for the detection of ovarian cancer had perfect specificity, low cost of implementation, and could lead to highly effective treatment, we would be quite willing to employ it as a means of saving the lives of just SOME women otherwise destined to die of this disease.

Question 7.22 In case-control studies of the efficacy of cancer screening, the receipt of the screening modality in question is ascertained in persons who sustained the outcome that screening sought to prevent (e.g., cancer mortality) during a period of time prior to diagnosis in which it is suspected that an abnormality would have been detectable via the screening test. Similar information is obtained from controls, typically persons at risk of the cancer being studied.

A critic of the above approach was concerned that "a screening test protects no one," but rather "the treatment that follows a test which is truly positive." He recommended as an alternative approach "a comparison of the previous frequency of *positive* screening tests leading to treatment of disease or preclinical states in cases and controls."

Do you agree with this recommendation? If yes, why do you agree? If not, why not?

Answer 7.22 Perhaps the best way to approach this question is by analogy to randomized trials of cancer screening efficacy. In such trials, we are trying to obtain information that will bear on the decision to recommend that a screening test be done, not that a POSITIVE test be done. Therefore, in the analysis of randomized trials of screening efficacy, the occurrence of cancer mortality is compared between persons offered and not offered screening; no attention is paid to the result, positive or negative, of a given test. Because the goal of a case-control study of screening efficacy is the same, the measure of "exposure" should be similar as well—the presence of screening in a particular subject, irrespective of the result.[58]

The fact is that positive screens would almost certainly be far more common in cases who died of the cancer than controls no matter what the efficacy (suggesting a harm from screening), given that all of the cases and virtually none of the controls would at some point prior to diagnosis have had pathology that (had a screening test been done) would have given rise to a positive result.

REFERENCES

1. Prescott E, Hippe M, Schnohr P, et al. Smoking and the risk of myocardial infarction in women and men: longitudinal population study. BMJ 1998;316:1043–6.
2. Kendal WS. Suicide and cancer: A gender-comparative study. Ann Oncol 2007;18:381–7.
3. Andriole GL, Crawford ED, Grubb RL, et al. Mortality results from a randomized prostate-cancer screening trial. N Engl J Med 2009;360:1310–9.
4. Carroll-Pankhurst C, Mortimer EA. Sudden infant death syndrome, bedsharing, parental weight, and age at death. Pediatrics 2001;107:530–6.
5. Kumar AS, Benz CC, Shim V, et al. Estrogen receptor-negative breast cancer is less likely to arise among lipophilic statin users. Cancer Epidemiol Biomarkers Prev 2008;17:1028–33.
6. Mosley BS, Cleves MA, Siega-Riz AM, et al. Neural tube defects and maternal folate intake among pregnancies conceived after folic acid fortification in the United States. Am J Epidemiol 2009;169:9–17.
7. Wong YN, Mitra N, Hudes G, et al. Survival associated with treatment vs observation of localized prostate cancer in elderly men. JAMA 2006;296:2683–93.

8. Christensen J, Gronborg TK, Sorensen MJ, et al. Prenatal valproate exposure and risk of autism spectrum disorders and childhood autism. JAMA 2013;309:1696–1703.

9. Galea S, Blaney S, Nandi A, et al. Explaining racial disparities in incidence of and survival from out-of-hospital cardiac arrest. Am J Epidemiol 2007;166:534–43.

10. Stromberg, B, Dahlquist G, Ericson A, et al. Neurological sequelae in children born after in-vitro fertilisation: a population-based study. Lancet 2002;359:461–5.

11. Weiss NS, Koepsell TD. Epidemiologic Methods. 2nd ed. New York: Oxford; 2014.

12. Hulley S, Grady D, Bush T, et al. Randomized trial of estrogen plus progestin for secondary prevention of coronary heart disease in postmenopausal women. JAMA 1998;280:605–13.

13. Cardo DM, Culver DH, Ciesielski CA, et al. A case-control study of seroconversion in health care workers. Centers for Disease Control and Prevention Needlestick Surveillance Group. N Engl J Med 1997;337:1485–90.

14. Steinmaus C, Yuan Y, Bates MN, et al. Case-control study of bladder cancer and drinking water arsenic in the western United States. Am J Epidemiol 2003;158:1193–201.

15. Furness S, Connor J, Robinson E, et al. Car colour and risk of car crash injury: population based case control study. BMJ 2003;327:1455–6.

16. Ray JG, Meier C, Vermeulen MJ, et al. Association of neural tube defects and folic acid food fortification in Canada. Lancet 2002;360:2047–8.

17. Lemaitre RN, Siscovick DS, Raghunathan TE, et al. Leisure-time physical activity and the risk of primary cardiac arrest. Arch Int Med 1999;159:686–90.

18. Jick SS, Hagberg KW, Kaye JA, et al. Postmenopausal estrogen-containing hormone therapy and the risk of breast cancer. Obstet Gynecol 2009;113:74–80.

19. Skjaerven R, Wilcox AJ, Lie RT. The interval between pregnancies and the risk of preeclampsia. N Engl J Med 2002;346:33–8.

20. Villeneuve PJ, Holowaty EJ, Brisson J, et al. Mortality among Canadian women with cosmetic breast implants. Am J Epidemiol 2006;164:334–41.

21. Pasternack B, Svanstrom H, Molgaard-Nielsen, et al. Metoclopramide in pregnancy and risk of major congenital malformations and fetal death. JAMA 2013;310:1601–11.
22. Nichol KL, Baken L, Wuorenma J, et al. The health and economic benefits associated with pneumococcal vaccination of elderly persons with chronic lung disease. Arch Intern Med 1999;159:2437–42.
23. Leonard RC, Kreckmann KH, Sakr CJ, et al. Retrospective cohort mortality study of workers in a polymer production plant including a reference population of regional workers. Ann Epidemiol 2008;18:15–22.
24. Stattin, P, Holmberg, E, Johansson, JE, et al. Outcomes in localized prostate cancer: National Prostate Cancer Register of Sweden followup study. J Nat Cancer Inst 2010;102:950–8.
25. Anderson JP, Ross JA, Folsom AR. Anthropometric variables, physical activity, and incidence of ovarian cancer. Cancer 2004;100:1515–21.
26. Beral V, Million Women Study Collaborators. Breast cancer and hormone-replacement therapy in the Million Women Study. Lancet 2003;362:419–27.
27. Youakim S. Risk of cancer among firefighters: a quantitative review of selected malignancies. Arch Environ Occup Health 2006;61:223–31.
28. Weiss NS, Rossing MA. Healthy screenee bias in epidemiologic studies of cancer incidence. Epidemiology 1996;7:319–22.
29. Caughey AB, Nicholson JM, Cheng YW, et al. Induction of labor and cesarean delivery by gestational age. Am J Obstet Gynecol 2006;195:700–5.
30. Chiazze L, Ference LD, Wolf PH: Mortality among automobile assembly workers: I. Spray painters. J Occup Med 1984;22:520–6.
31. Collins S, Ramsay M, Slack MPE, et al. Risk of invasive Haemophilus influenza infection during pregnancy and association with adverse fetal outcomes. JAMA 2014;311:1125–32.
32. Rowe B, Milner R, Johnson C, et al. The association of alcohol and night driving with fatal snowmobile injury: a case-control study. Ann Emerg Med 1994;24:842–8.

33. Heffelfinger JD, Heckbert SR, Psaty BM, et al. Influenza vaccination and risk of incident myocardial infarction. Hum Vaccin 2006;2:161–6.

34. Spirtas R, Heineman EF, Bernstein L, et al. Malignant mesothelioma: Attributable risk of asbestos exposure. Occup Environ Med 1994;51:804–11.

35. Rosenberg L, Rao RS, Palmer JR, et al. Transitional cell cancer of the urinary tract and renal cell cancer in relation to acetaminophen use. Cancer Causes Control 1998;9:83–8.

36. Handke M, Harloff A, Olschewski M, et al. Patent foramen ovale and cryptogenic stroke in older patients. N Engl J Med. 2007;351:2262–8.

37. Hessel PA, Teta MJ, Goodman M, et al. Mesothelioma among brake mechanics: an expanded analysis of a case-control study. Risk Anal 2004;24:547–52.

38. Asbridge M, Mann R, Cusimano MD, et al. Cannabis and traffic collision risk: findings from a case-crossover study of injured drivers presenting to emergency departments. Int J Public Health 2014;59:395–404.

39. Grant AM, Avenell A, Campbell MK, et al. Oral vitamin D3 and calcium for secondary prevention of low-trauma fractures in elderly people: a randomised placebo-controlled trial. Lancet 2005;365:1621–8.

40. Glynn RJ, Danielson E, Fonseca FA, et al. A randomized trial of rosuvastatin in the prevention of venous thromboembolism. N Engl J Med 2009;360:1851–61.

41. John EM, Koo J, Horn-Ross PL. Lifetime physical activity and risk of endometrial cancer. Cancer Epidemiol Biomarkers Prev 2010;19:1276–83.

42. Donnell D, Baeten JM, Kiarie J, et al. Heterosexual HIV-1 transmission after initiation of antiretroviral therapy: a prospective cohort analysis. Lancet 2010;375:2092–8.

43. Treggiari MM, Weiss NS. Occupational asbestos exposure and the incidence of non-Hodgkin lymphoma of the gastrointestinal tract: an ecologic study. Ann Epidemiol 2004;14:168–71.

44. Yuan JM, Gao YT, Ong CN, et al. Prediagnostic level of serum retinol in relation to reduced risk of hepatocellular carcinoma. J Natl Cancer Inst 2006;98:482–90.

45. Palefsky JM, Giuliano AR, Goldstone S, et al. HPV vaccine against anal HPV infection and anal intraepithelial neoplasia. N Engl J Med 2011;365:1576–85.

46. Nevadunsky NS, Van Arsdale A, Strickler HD, et al. Obesity and age at diagnosis of endometrial cancer. Obstet Gynecol 2014;124:300–6.

47. Keall MD, Pierse N, Howden-Chapman P, et al. Home modifications to reduce injuries from falls in the Home Injury Prevention Intervention Study: a cluster-randomized controlled trial. Lancet 2015;385:231–8.

48. McPherson CP, Swenson KK, Jolitz G, et al. Survival of women ages 40–49 years with breast carcinoma according to method of detection. Cancer 1997;79:1923–32.

49. Fenton JJ, Taplin SH, Carney PA, et al. Influence of computer-aided detection on performance of screening mammography. N Engl J Med 2007;356:1399–1409.

50. Mandel JS, Church TR, Ederer F, et al. Colorectal cancer mortality: effectiveness of biennial screening for fecal occult blood. J Natl Cancer Inst 1999;91:434–7.

51. Yang B, Morrell S, Zuo Y, et al. A case-control study of the protective benefit of cervical screening against invasive cervical cancer in NSW women. Cancer Causes Control 2008;19:569–76.

52. Hackam DG, Thiruchelvam D, Redelmeier DA. Angiotensin-converting enzyme inhibitors and aortic rupture: a population-based case-control study. Lancet 2006; 368:659–65.

53. Bergstralh EJ, Roberts RO, Farmer SA, et al. Population-based case-control study of PSA and DRE screening on prostate cancer mortality. Urology 2007;70:936–41.

54. Rustin GJ, van der Burg ME, Griffin CL, et al. Early versus delayed treatment of relapsed ovarian cancer. Lancet 2010;376:1155–63.

55. Weiss NS. Control definition in case-control studies of the efficacy of screening and diagnostic testing. Am J Epidemiol 1983;118:457–60.

56. Thompson SG, Ashton HA, Gao L, Scott RA. Screening men for abdominal aortic aneurysm: 10 year mortality and cost effectiveness results from the randomised Multicentre Aneurysm Screening Study. BMJ 2009;338:b2307.

57. Weiss NS, Dhillon PK, Etzioni RS. Case-control studies of the efficacy of cancer screening. Overcoming bias from nonrandom patterns of screening. Epidemiology 2004;15:409–13.
58. Weiss NS. Case-control studies of screening: A response to George Knox. Public Health 1992;106:127–30.